MW01230029

NOURISH

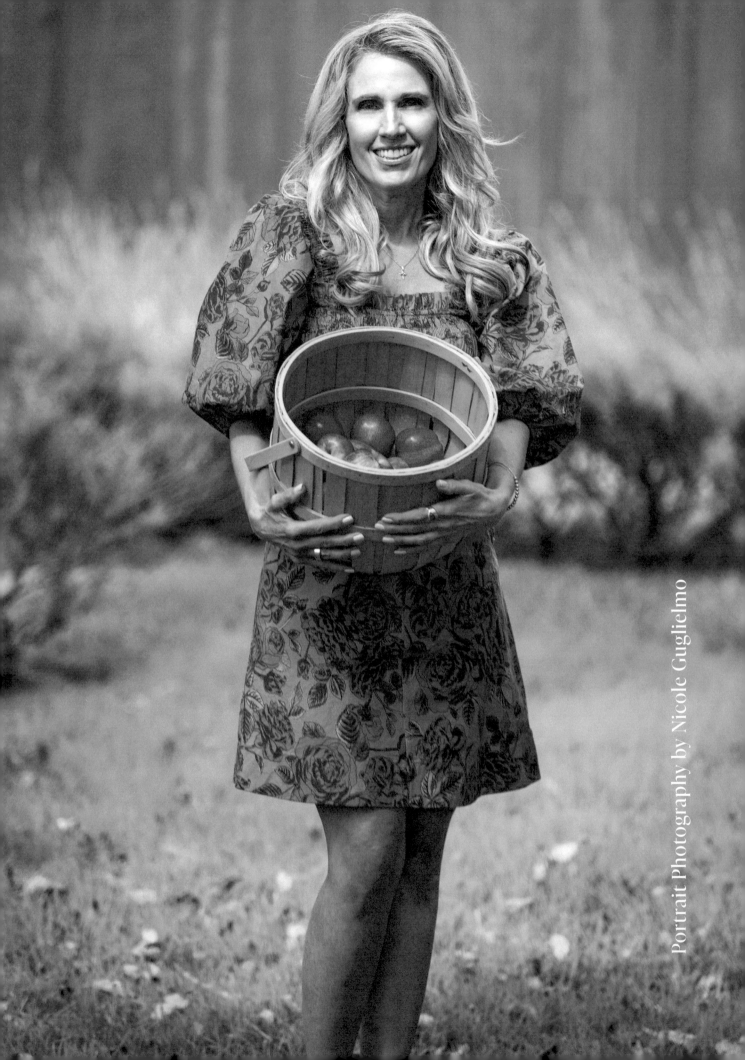

NOURISH

Celebrating Nature's Harvest
& A Healthy Lifestyle

MARY ABITANTO

Author of *Food That Will Gather Your Family,*
Food From My Heart & Home, and *Gather For The Holidays*

Contributing Editor:

SAMARA KRAFT, MS, RDN, CDCES

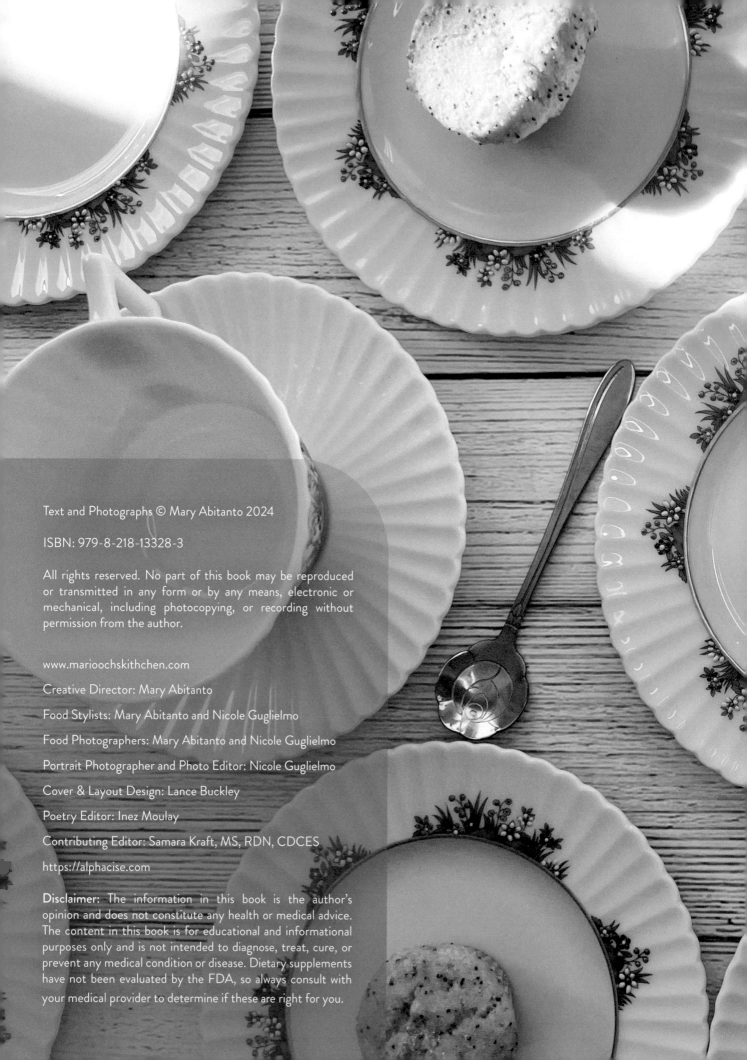

www.marioochskithchen.com

Creative Director: Mary Abitanto

Food Stylists: Mary Abitanto and Nicole Guglielmo

Food Photographers: Mary Abitanto and Nicole Guglielmo

Portrait Photographer and Photo Editor: Nicole Guglielmo

Cover & Layout Design: Lance Buckley

Poetry Editor: Inez Moulay

Contributing Editor: Samara Kraft, MS, RDN, CDCES

https://alphacise.com

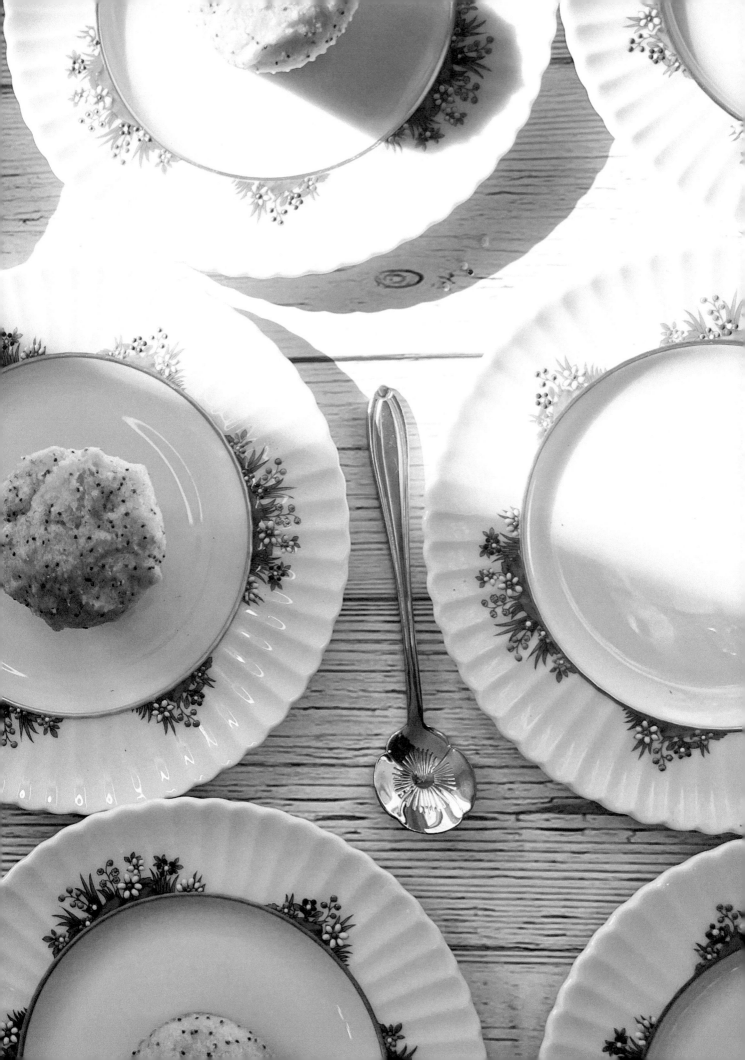

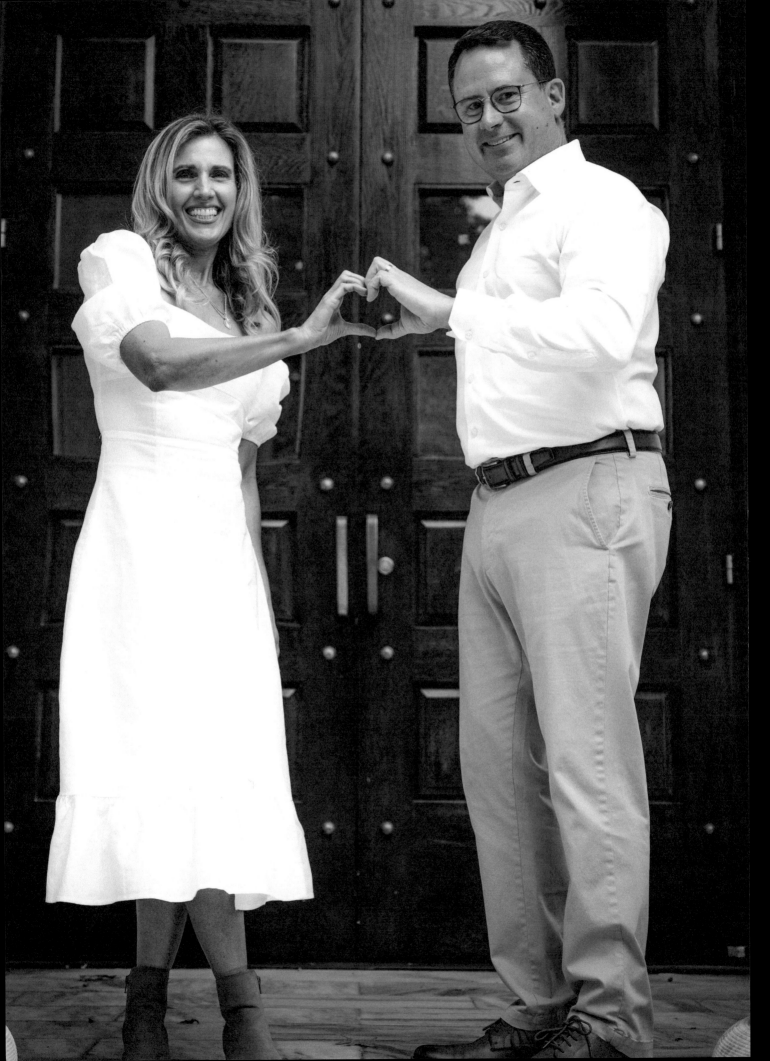

DEDICATION

This book is dedicated to my beloved parents, Midge and Mike. I am eternally grateful for the invaluable life lessons they have taught me by their quiet and steady example of hard work, love, and steadfast faith in God. Being their daughter was a true blessing in my life.

I have such fond memories of working with Mom side by side in the garden, spring through summer. She taught me how to stake out the garden, till the soil, plant the garden, plant marigolds to repel any little critters, and of course, there was the weeding, not a particular joy, but nonetheless I did it.

Reaping the benefits of my hard work was something I learned at a very early age. Now, I share my love of gardening with my children, and we care for our own garden which for some years has just been a planter filled with fresh basil. These days it's a larger garden in a lovely wood-crafted raised bed that my landscaper built for me. If you don't have the space, I encourage you to cultivate your own garden, even if it's in a small planter. If the planter is large enough you can grow eggplants, try it! Always consider the quality of the soil and if it is contaminated with pesticides before you plant it in the ground, a raised bed might be a better option as well as purchasing fresh organic soil to fill it.

My memories with Dad, as it relates to this book, are connected to enjoying fresh produce. His first job, at age five, was as a peddler of fruits and vegetables, I suppose our family has a stellar work ethic. He taught me how to test for the freshest and most ripe cantaloupe and fruit. Cutting up a pineapple was a particular talent of his, and one which I learned. He shared with me his love for fresh black mission figs, which we would indulge in every summer at the local farmer's market in a quaint little fishing village in our cozy beach town. It was something I looked forward to every summer. The long-awaited bite into a ripened and juicy, red-fleshed fig–Oh how I love that taste.

When Dad was in the U. S. Army, he was a big fan of peppers and eggs. He would always tell the story that where he was stationed there was no butter, but an abundance of eggs from the chickens and peppers from the local farms, so he would enjoy a pepper and egg sandwich with mayonnaise.

In our garden, we planted peppers, eggplant, and tomatoes every spring. If you have my other books, you know how much I love eggplant. Pop was the Italian chef extraordinaire in the family and made the best eggplant parmesan from our harvested eggplants. He truly loved all vegetables, and this love of fresh produce (and Italian cooking) was bestowed onto me and is now being celebrated in this book.

> *Thank you to those of you who have served our country. We are grateful for your service. My father served in the U.S. Army and was stationed in Panama. After his service, he went to college at the University of Maryland on the G.I. Bill and completed a master's degree. The Army instilled so many valuable lessons which my father incorporated into his way of life. One glance at his shiny, polished shoes, and you knew he had been in the Army. He was always properly dressed.*

It has come full circle, because now my children and I make delicious recipes from my garden gatherings. My daughter Maggie and I have been making pickled cucumbers and onions and we share the recipes in this book. My son Jack and I experiment often with the basil from the garden and make all kinds of pesto combinations: spinach and basil pesto, parsley and basil pesto, and arugula and basil pesto. We omit the nuts because Jack and my husband, Peter, are allergic, so we make it an herbed pesto and it's so good. We share a recipe in this book. My daughter Sydney and I love making fresh apple pie come fall, sometimes we are lucky to use our own apples. In this book, we share a very special baked oatmeal recipe with tiny bite-sized apples. It is my go-to breakfast topped with maple syrup.

The eggplant in my garden blooms very late in the season. I will still pick them as late as September. I have an abundance of recipes using eggplant and share a few in this book. They are all gluten-free.

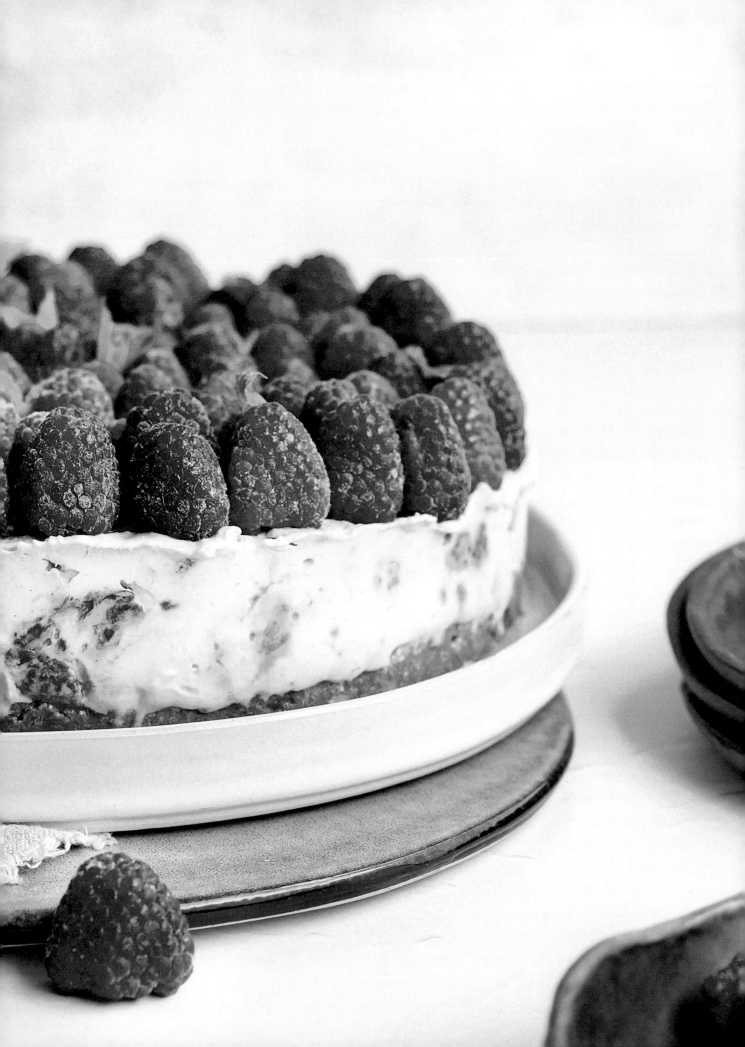

MY DEEPEST GRATITUDE

There are a lot of moving parts and people involved in writing a book. You can only imagine all the components that go into it. Conceptualizing the idea, creating the recipes, testing the recipes, food styling, food photographs, editing, book layout and design, and finally marketing the book.

As always, I am so grateful to those of you who follow my cooking journey, which is really my life's journey. Thank you for picking up my book(s), being so excited to read them, and sending me notes, texts, and detailed letters pouring out your love for my books (and recipes!). As always, don't forget to write a review on amazon if you love the book. That is tremendously helpful to me.

I am so blessed to have an amazing photographer, Nicole. She is also a very talented food stylist and took a few food photos in this book. I am eternally grateful to her for her enthusiasm for my work and her excitement to see the outcome.

My sister Irene was helpful with reading my poetry and encouraging me to add more to this book. Robert Frost said that poetry should be "Like a piece of ice on a hot stove the poem must ride on its own melting."[1] If you write poetry, keep that in mind. It can flow as you wish it to flow, like a river. Irene was also very helpful with content and chapter layout. I am so blessed to have a sister who is also my own personal cheerleader.

I am deeply grateful to my friend Samara, a nutritionist, who weighs in on eating healthy, diet trends, maintaining heart and brain health, and other wellness tips at the end of this book. Her expertise in this field is unsurpassed and her knowledge is impressive. You will all benefit from her insight.

My friend Sharon helped me recipe test a few of the recipes in this book and my other books. She also gave me input on content and chapter layout. I am

so grateful to her for her kindness and willingness to help me amid a busy life of being a mom, grandma, a dog mom, and caring for her family.

My taste testers were in abundance for this book. Being that I had developed many gluten-free recipes, I especially needed taste testers who are familiar with gluten-free baking and cooking. My niece Kristen was one of those testers. She is always so enthusiastic and impressed with what gluten-free recipes I am churning out in my kitchen. I am so grateful for her kindness and enthusiasm.

My friend and neighbor Adriana was another person who I would run to with a finished dessert or bread, typically not gluten free. She has lived and traveled all over the world, so I value her opinion and I am grateful for her input.

My friend and neighbor John, who has multiple degrees including a Doctorate in Synthetic Organic Chemistry from UC Berkeley, was very helpful teaching me about food science. I am so grateful for his willingness to help me understand (and then apply) the science behind gluten-free baking. It was like being a student in an accelerated chemistry course. A huge thank you!

Thank you to my friends including Chef Rosangela who graciously shared a recipe in this book and gave me feedback on some of my recipes, and other friends who gave me input regarding my cover and recipes. Their enthusiasm and kindness are deeply appreciated.

Last but not least thank you to my family and my kids' friends who were all so helpful with giving their input on recipes they tasted. Keep in mind, my family will only tell me its good, if it's good. All the recipes in this book passed their taste testing. My brother Michael gave my coffee cake a thumbs up!

---

[1]Source: Robert Frost. The Figure a Poem Makes (1939)

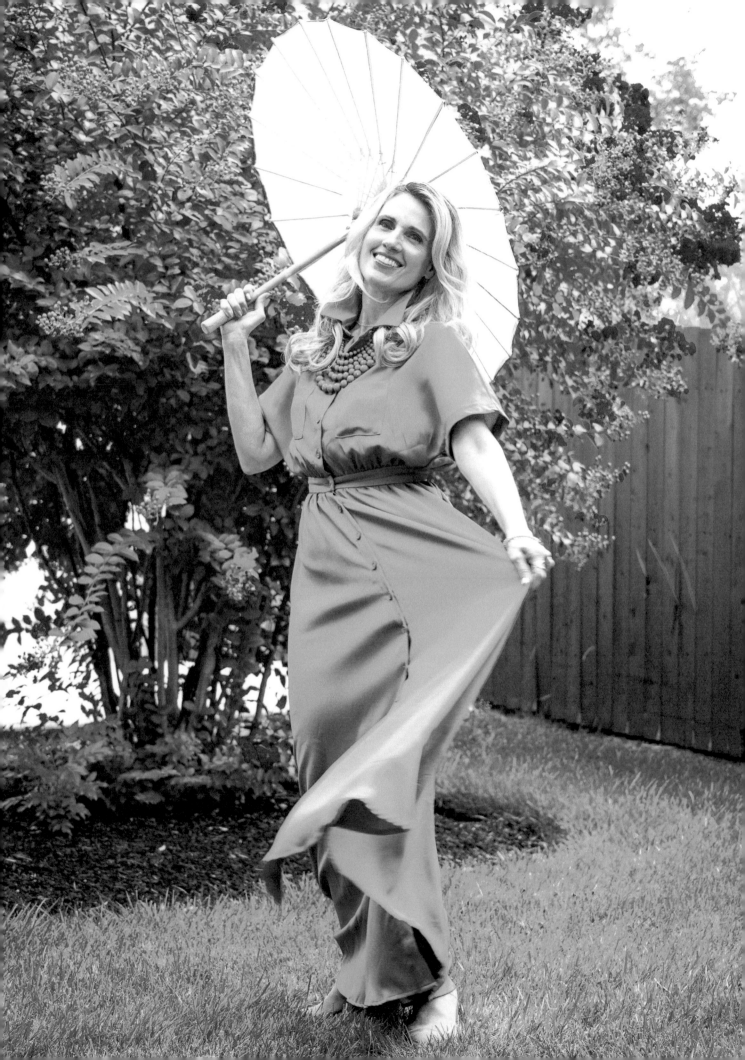

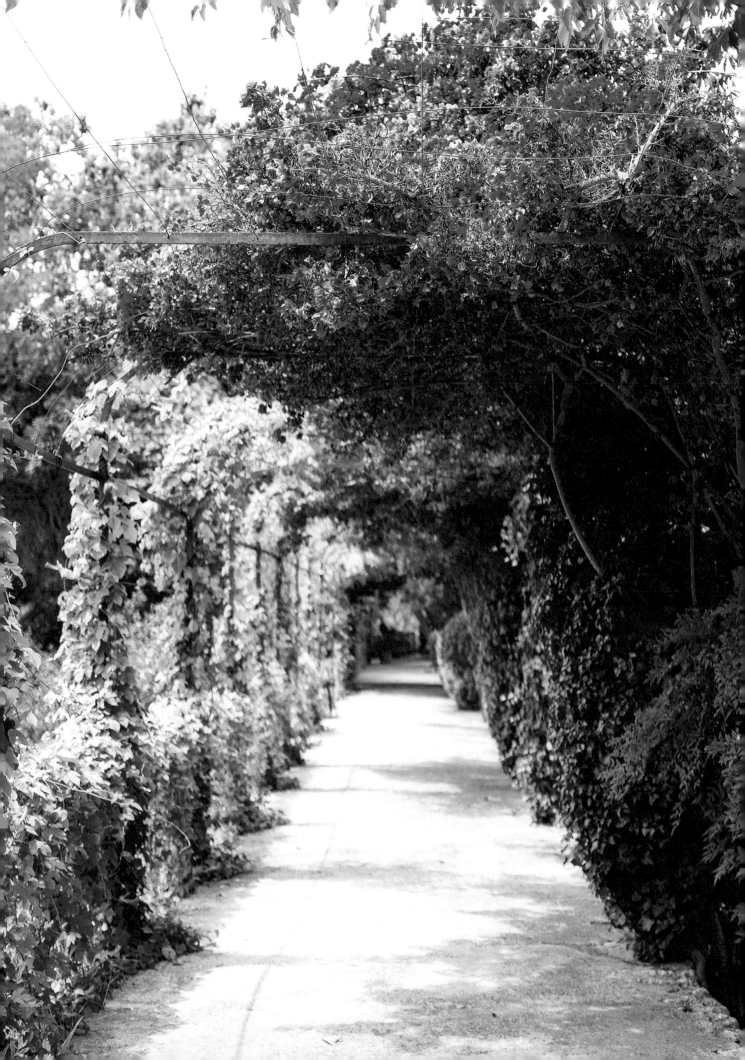

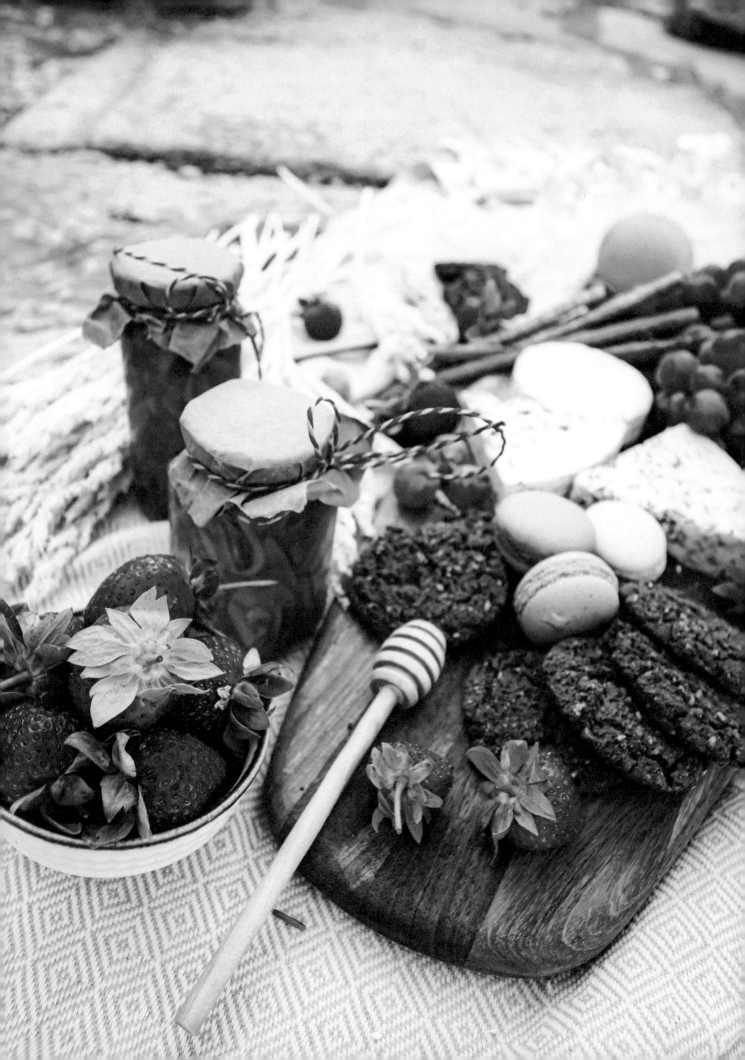

INTRODUCTION

Welcome to my kitchen. It is always a pleasure picking up right where I left off with my other books. If you have my cookbooks, you know that my specialty as a home chef is feeding the family healthy meals. My house feels like a revolving door for friends and family. If you want the kids to hang around your house, learn how to cook. It's as simple as that.

NOURISH is the overarching theme of this cookbook. I encourage you to nourish your family, friends, and yourselves through good nutrition and by incorporating more fruit, vegetables, herbs, and legumes like beans, chick peas, and lentils into your diet. Eating healthy will give you more sustainable energy to do the things you love. Living a healthy lifestyle is about eating wholesome and nutritious foods most of the time, while still enjoying the foods you love. In this book, we turn to nature's harvest to inspire our recipes and teach our palate to eat more healthfully. However, we can still enjoy bread, pizza, pasta, cake, and cookies which are also included in this book. It's about striking a balance. Although this is not a gluten-free cookbook, it has plenty of gluten-free recipes like bagels, pizzas, gnocchi, cakes, muffins, and cookies. Most recipes in this book are adaptable to a gluten-free lifestyle. It's the book where the gluten-free world and gluten world live harmoniously.

Today's families have mixed dietary needs. Some family members may be living a gluten-free lifestyle like my daughter Maggie does from time to time; others like to indulge in bread and pasta, like my son Jack and daughter Sydney; others are vegetarians or just prefer eating less meat. I fall into the category of eating more vegetable-based meals, legumes, and less meat. I am living a Mediterranean lifestyle. Nutritionist Samara Kraft talks more about the benefits of a Mediterranean-style diet in the Q & A section at the end of this book. Regardless, I think we can all agree that most families have a mix of eating styles that they must accommodate for their

meal planning. This book will be your go-to guide for family meal planning.

With my newest cookbook, *NOURISH Celebrating Nature's Harvest & A Healthy Lifestyle,* I want to be sure it is inclusive, and that it not only meets but surpasses the needs of a gluten-free lifestyle. I wanted to blow it out of the park, so to speak. You can have your cake and eat it too. Pun intended. I also make adaptations for a vegetarian lifestyle when possible; however, there are still meat recipes included in this book.

A little back story. If you read my first cookbook, *Food That Will Gather Your Family,* you will know that when my son Jack was 10 months old, he was diagnosed with multiple food allergies. Wheat and barley were two of them and avoiding gluten was something we did for years. I developed recipes that avoided gluten, but the challenge was to create the best-tasting recipes as well, because I didn't want Jack to miss out. At that time, he was allergic to forty different allergens! Yes, you read that right. The task was indeed momentous, but my will was strong. I wanted Jack to eat the best food, and the quest began. I made gluten-free bread, pasta, cookies, cakes, and so much more. Jack's food allergy was the catalyst that started me cooking in my kitchen. Developing gluten-free recipes was something I was good at and enjoyed doing. He has since outgrown his allergy to wheat and barley.

Fast forward, seventeen years later, and many people today are living a gluten-free lifestyle either by choice because it makes them feel better, or due to an allergy or Celiac's Disease. This is the first time that I am sharing my recipe ideas in the gluten-free realm in a cookbook alongside my other recipes which contain gluten.

Thankfully, the gluten-free flour options are in abundance today. When I reached out to Bob's

Red Mill about developing gluten-free recipes for my newest cookbook, they graciously sent me a good variety of their gluten-free flours for my recipe testing. I am grateful for their kindness. I use Super-Fine Almond Flour by Bob's Red Mill for all my baking recipes that include almond flour. Whatever brand you choose, however, be sure that you are using a super-fine blend of almond flour otherwise the outcome of the recipe may be unpredictable. It's important to note that ground flaxseed is also known as flax meal. I use flax meal in some of my recipes.

I also reached out to King Arthur Baking Company, and they, too, sent me a nice variety of products. One which I love is their Gluten-Free Measure for Measure Flour. It was such a kind gesture and so appreciated.

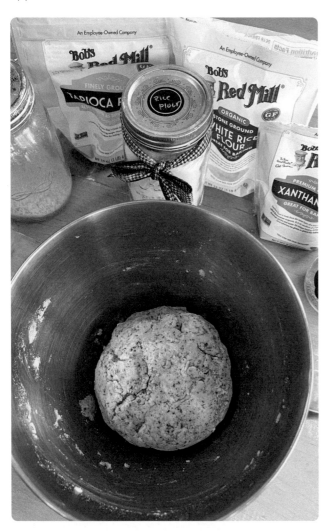

I worked tirelessly creating many gluten-free recipes that have been tested, retested, and taste-tested by some gluten-free critics. I have identified a need and realize people struggle finding good-tasting gluten-free bagels, pizzas, pasta, cakes, muffins, and cookies. With a little fancy footwork and a little food science, I have included those in this book along with other recipes containing gluten–most of which can be adapted to be gluten free with some minor adjustments, like switching flours. If so, I will mention the adaptation within the recipe. There are *plenty* of gluten-free options in this book that you will not only like but truly fall in love with. The truth is that they are so good that even those who do not live a gluten-free lifestyle will enjoy them. My gluten-free bagels will be loved by everyone!

The pages of this book brim with a vast collection of recipes that will please the palate. All my recipes are paired with stunning photographs taken by yours truly (and a few by Nicole) to capture your eye and steal your heart. You will fall in love with the recipes on these pages.

I've also included a photo of Mom's storied china, a cherished family heirloom. Every holiday when I take it out, I am reminded to celebrate life and enjoy good food. There is a small collection of eloquent poetry, inspired by nature's harvest in all its glory. And yes, for those of you who know me, there is a picture of the horses which I live close to. Every day I get to see the gallant horse's trot. At the very end of the book, my friend Samara Kraft, a nutritionist, weighs in on eating healthy, diet trends, maintaining heart and brain health, and other wellness tips. You won't want to put the book down.

This book is a celebration of nature's harvest intended to inspire you and your family for generations to come. Pull up a chair, pour a cup of coffee, matcha tea, or double espresso, if you dare, and indulge in a book that may change the way you eat and think about food. Nature's bounty awaits you! Let's get started on the most delicious food journey of your life. . .

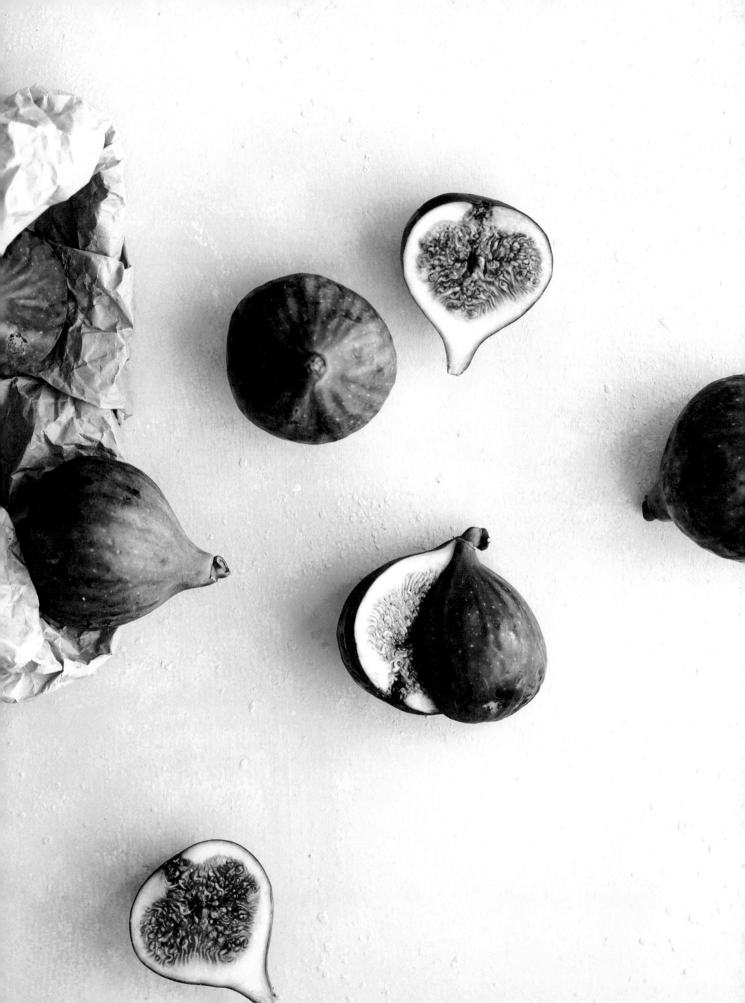

CONTENTS

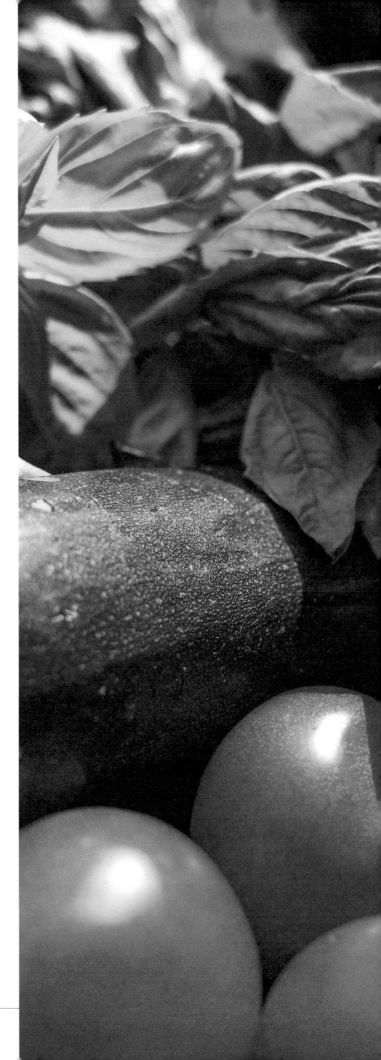

PASTA, POTATO DUMPLINGS, AND SAUCES

PIZZAS AND BREADS

DESSERTS

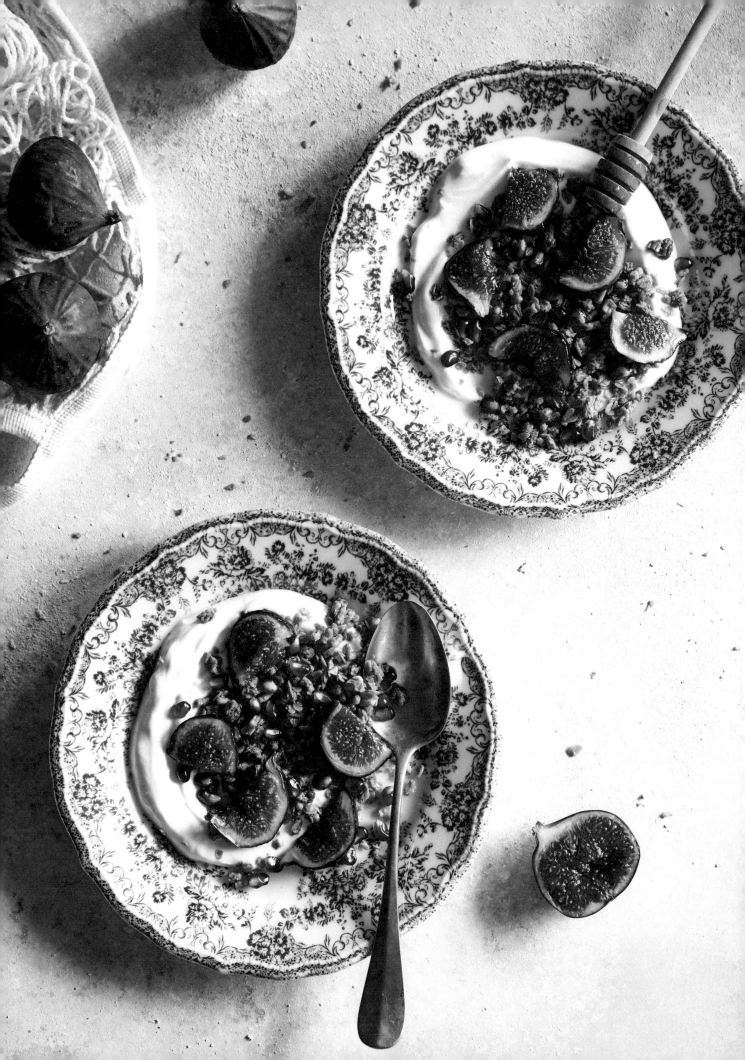

SWEET MORNINGS

COFFEE CAKE

DOGELS

STRAWBERRY OAT BITES
(Gluten Free)

SHAKES

BAKED OATMEAL WITH APPLES
(Gluten Free)

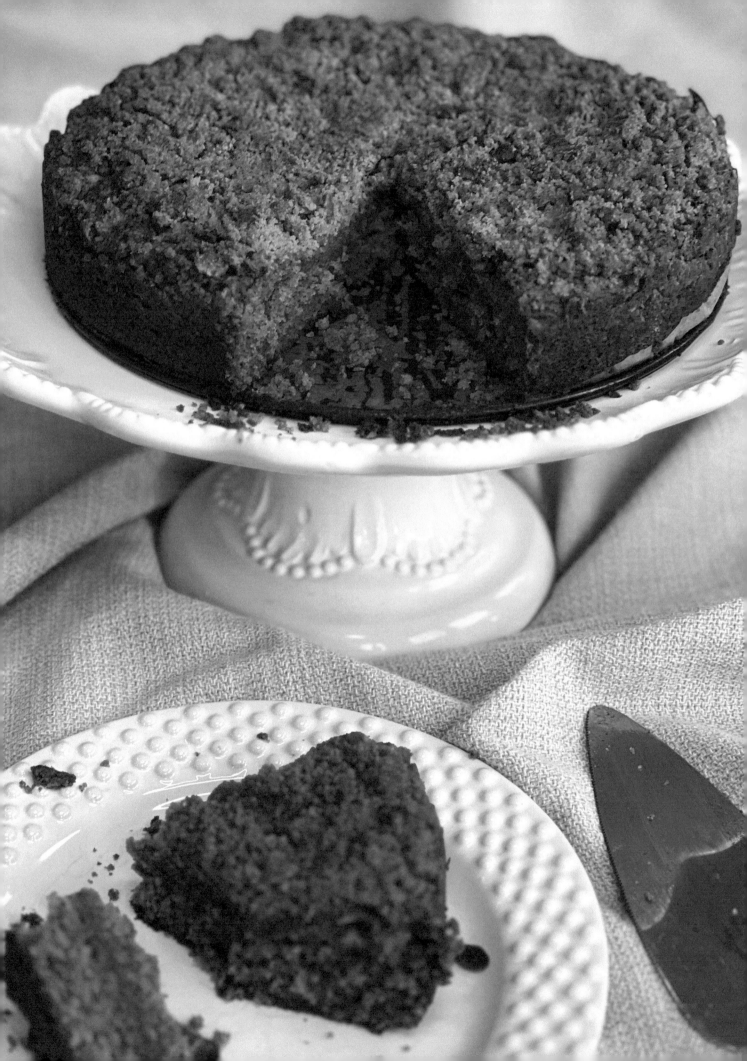

COFFEE CAKE
SERVES 8

Living a healthy lifestyle is about eating wholesome and nutritious foods most of the time, while still enjoying the foods you love. With that said, this is a fabulous coffee cake recipe, that I made a healthy swap for olive oil instead of butter for the inside of the cake. The topping, however, contains butter to make it that crunchy, buttery texture you would expect from a quintessential streusel topping.

Enjoy a slice with a hot cup of coffee for a sweet treat. In the summer, you can add a handful of fresh blueberries to the top of the cake. Swap pumpkin purée in lieu of sour cream to give this cake a fall update. It's an adaptable recipe that everyone will love. An easy swap to make this gluten free is to swap out the flour for gluten-free flour: King Arthur Baking Company's Gluten-Free Measure For Measure Flour is a good choice.

INGREDIENTS

- ½ cup light brown sugar, packed
- ½ cup granulated sugar
- 1 cup sour cream, room temperature
- 1 cup extra virgin olive oil
- 1–2 teaspoons vanilla extract
- 2 large eggs, room temperature
- 2 cups all-purpose flour (or cake flour, or gluten-free flour), spooned and leveled
- 1 teaspoon baking soda
- 1 teaspoon baking powder
- 1 tablespoon cinnamon
- ¼ teaspoon cardamom
- ¼ teaspoon salt
- ½ cup powdered sugar for dusting cake (optional)
- Stand mixer with paddle attachment (or hand mixer)
- 9-inch springform pan

Streusel Topping:

- 1 cup all-purpose flour (or gluten-free flour)
- ¾ cup light brown sugar, packed
- 2 ½ teaspoons cinnamon
- ⅛ teaspoon cardamon spice
- 1 stick salted butter, softened

Cinnamon-Brown Sugar Topping:

- ¼ cup light brown sugar
- 2 teaspoons cinnamon

OPTIONAL:

Icing:

- ½ cup powdered sugar
- 3 teaspoons milk

Preheat the oven to 350 degrees.

In the bowl of the stand mixer, add the brown sugar and mix on low to break up any chunks. Then add the granulated sugar, sour cream, olive oil, and vanilla. Mix on medium speed until all the ingredients are well combined. Then stream in the premixed eggs and mix on medium until well combined. Do not over mix.

Baking tip: Always spoon the flour into a measuring cup and then level it off for the most accurate measurement for any of my baking recipes. Scooping up the flour will firmly pack it into the measuring cup and add more than needed, creating a denser outcome.

In a small bowl, add the flour, baking soda, baking powder, cinnamon, and cardamom, and whisk. Then add the dry ingredients to the wet ingredients. Mix on medium speed until the batter is smooth.

A tip on loosening hardened brown sugar is to add a slice of bread (or gluten-free bread) to the container and leave it overnight. In the morning, it will be completely unhardened and have a sand-like texture.

Note: If you use gluten-free flour be sure it includes xanthan gum in the ingredient listing–if it doesn't, add ½ teaspoon to this cake. You may experience different baking results depending on the gluten-free flour blend you choose.

Prepare the springform pan by adding butter to the sides of the pan along with a dusting of flour. Next, cut out a circle of parchment paper to fit inside the bottom of the pan.

Make the Cinnamon-Brown Sugar Topping.

Combine the ingredients in a small bowl and mix with a fork or whisk. Set this aside.

Make the Streusel Topping.

Combine the dry ingredients in a bowl and mix with a fork to get out any lumps. Next, melt the butter for 28–29 seconds in a microwave-safe bowl in the microwave and add it to the dry ingredients. Mix until you have achieved a crumbly texture. Use your hands to break it up into bits. Alternatively, you may use a food processor and pulse until you have coarse crumbs.

> Note: Feel free to double the streusel topping ingredients to get a higher crumb topping.

To the springform pan, add half of the batter and tap on the counter to spread it evenly. Combine the brown sugar and cinnamon and sprinkle on top. Then add the remaining batter and spread with a spoon or a spatula to evenly distribute it. Last, layer with the streusel topping.

Bake for 45–50 minutes. It's done once a toothpick comes out clean in the center of the cake and it springs back. Oven temperatures may vary.

Allow the cake to cool for 30 minutes, then release it from the pan. Allow the cake to cool on the cooling rack for an additional 30 minutes. Leave the bottom of the pan intact while cooling.

Make the Icing.

Whisk powdered sugar and milk until you have achieved a thick consistency.

Once cooled, transfer the cake to a cake stand by carefully releasing the bottom. Add a dusting of powdered sugar. Cut each slice and drizzle on the icing.

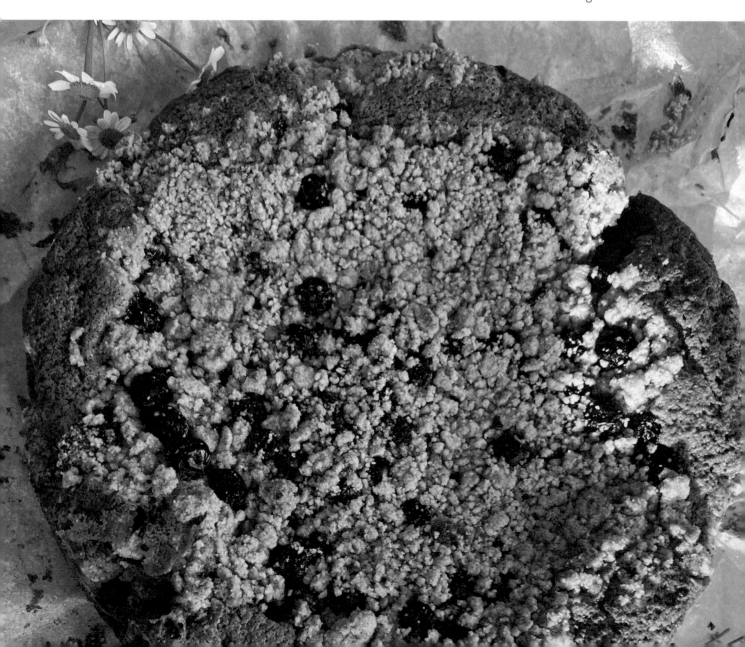

DOGELS

Donuts meet bagels in this tasty, sticky, twisted pastry bread ring dubbed a "Dogel" by my family. This will be your new weekend go-to breakfast treat. It's airy on the inside and baked to crunchy perfection, creating a beautiful cinnamon-sugar crust.

INGREDIENTS:

- 3 ½ cups all-purpose flour
- 1 packet rapid-rise yeast, or 2 ¼ teaspoons
- 1 ½ teaspoons table salt
- 4 tablespoons granulated sugar
- 4 tablespoons salted butter, softened
- 1 ⅛ cup low-fat milk
- A drizzle of olive oil
- Stand mixer with hook attachment
- Wood pastry board

Date Syrup:

- 6 medjool dates, pitted plus ½ cup water
- 1 ½ cups hot water
- Small pot
- Strainer or cheesecloth

Topping:

- 2 cups granulated sugar
- 4 tablespoons cinnamon

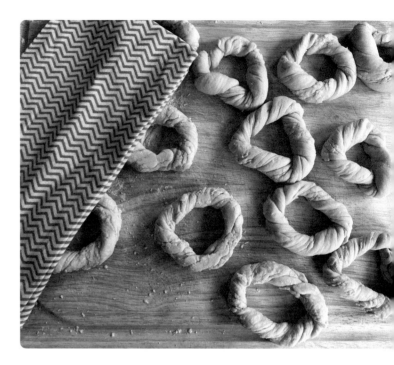

In the stand mixer bowl, combine the flour, yeast, salt, sugar, and butter. Next, mix on low and drizzle in the milk slowly until the dough starts to come together and pulls away from the sides of the bowl. If it's too sticky, add 1 tablespoon of flour at a time. Knead for 5 minutes to fully incorporate all the ingredients. The stand mixer will have done most of the work for you.

Next, add a tiny drizzle of oil to the stand mixer bowl. Add the dough and cover with a clean dish towel. Place in a warm spot to rise.

Make the Date Syrup.

Boil dates plus ½ cup water for 5 minutes until dates soften. Strain into a bowl, or once cooled, through a cheesecloth, catching all the liquid in a bowl. You can use the leftover dates (solids) in another recipe. Set the date liquid aside.

Once the dough has doubled in size, about 1 ½ hours, you can make the Dogels.

On a pastry board, cut the dough into 10 chunks. Roll each chunk into a long rope, about 10 inches long. Twist the dough on both ends in opposite directions, and then seal ends together forming a ring.

Make the Topping.

Combine 1 cup of sugar plus 2 tablespoons of cinnamon on a flat plate. Once the mixture gets too wet, discard and add the remaining 1 cup of sugar and 2 tablespoons of cinnamon.

Next, combine 1 ½ cups hot water with ½ cup of the strained date liquid. Dip the Dogels twice in the liquid, then dip the Dogels in the topping mixture.

Place the Dogels onto a parchment-lined baking sheet. Cover and allow them to puff up for 20 minutes. If there is any liquid around the Dogels, soak it up with a paper towel.

Bake at 425 degrees for 17 minutes until golden brown, turn halfway through. These freeze well.

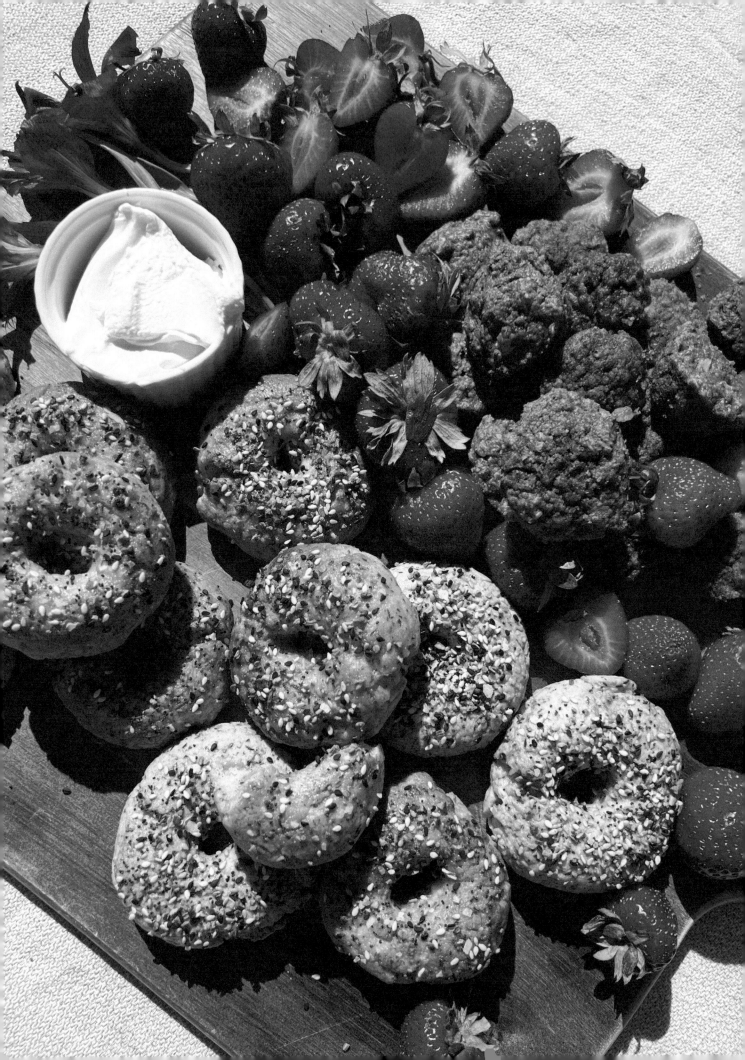

STRAWBERRY OAT BITES
(Gluten Free)

INGREDIENTS:

- 1 ½ cups halved fresh (or frozen) organic strawberries
- ¼ cup chopped dates (about 2-3 dates)
- ⅓ cup dark brown sugar
- ⅛ cup sugar-free maple syrup
- 1 cup plus 2 tablespoons olive oil
- 1 teaspoon vanilla extract
- 1 egg plus 1 egg yolk (or 1 flax egg, recipe follows)
- 2 cups gluten-free thick-cut organic whole oats, pulsed (I used Bob's Red Mill)
- ½ cup gluten-free thick-cut organic whole oats, not pulsed
- ½ teaspoon baking soda
- ½ teaspoon cinnamon
- ½ teaspoon xanthan gum
- Stand mixer with paddle attachment
- 24 mini-muffin tin
- Non-stick cooking spray
- High-speed blender

Preheat the oven to 350 degrees.

Note: If you are using frozen strawberries allow them to thaw completely, about 20 minutes or longer.

Add the dates to a cup of warm water so they become soft, then chop.

In the bowl of the stand mixer, add the fresh or thawed strawberries. Mix on medium speed until they start to break up. Add the chopped dates, sugar, maple syrup, olive oil, and vanilla. Mix on medium speed until they start to liquify. Last, drizzle in the premixed egg slowly and continue to mix until everything is well incorporated.

In the high-speed blender, add 2 cups of whole oats and pulse until they become powder-like. I used extra thick oats that measured 2 cups when pulsed. If you use regular oats, add a little more to the blender, then measure. Add them to a bowl along with ½ cup of whole oats and baking soda, cinnamon, and xanthan gum. Whisk until combined.

Add the dry ingredients to the wet ingredients and mix for 1 minute on medium speed, scraping down the sides and bottom of the bowl with a spatula.

Scoop up the batter, using a tablespoon, and fill the greased muffin tins with the batter. Bake for 14–15 minutes until slightly golden. These are pictured with my Everything Bagels (Gluten Free) (page 20).

Harvest tip: Blueberry and strawberry season runs from May to August in New Jersey. In some parts of the country, you can find berries as early as March or April. This is the best time of year to visit your local farmer's markets and take advantage of fresh produce. If you want to maximize the taste in this recipe, choose organic. Be inspired by what is fresh and in season, and cook your meals and desserts based on that.

Baker's tip: Thoroughly wash and dry fresh stawberries, cut off the stem, and place them onto a baking sheet and then into the freezer. Once frozen solid, place them into a freezer bag. This will preserve the nutrients and you will have strawberries to make this delicious recipe when you wish.

Flax egg is 1 tablespoon of ground flaxseed (or flax meal) plus 2 ½–3 tablespoons water. Mix and allow it to sit for 5 minutes. You may use this as a substitute in any recipe requiring 1 large egg. I use Bob's Red Mill Whole Ground Flaxseed Meal in my recipes.

GREEN MATCHA SHAKE

MAKES 2 SHAKES

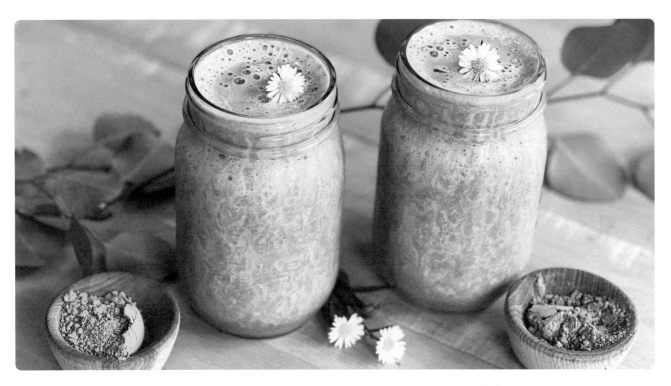

INREDIENTS:

- 1 teaspoon organic matcha powder
- 1 ½ cups nonfat milk (or milk alternative, almond, or oat milk)
- 2 small, ripened bananas
- ½ cup frozen organic spinach
- 1 tablespoon tahini
- 2 heaping tablespoons chocolate protein powder (or unflavored collagen powder)
- 1 tablespoon sugar-free maple syrup
- 1 teaspoon cacao powder (or cocoa powder)
- 1 teaspoon Organic Basil Seeds by Zen Basil (or chai seeds)
- Ice as needed
- 2 medium-sized mason jars
- Straws for sipping
- High-speed blender

Mix all ingredients in the blender until creamy. If it's too thick, add more milk. If it's too runny, add more ice.

You will love this so matcha!

Note: Matcha is a high-grade green tea ground into powder. It's best to use organic matcha powder if you can find it. It is produced without the use of pesticides or chemicals. Protein and collagen powders are recommended for adults, not kids. Consult with your pediatrician on any supplements.

Nutrition tip: Milk is a great source of calcium, but did you know that tahini which is made from ground sesame seeds is also a good source of calcium. It has a creamy and nutty profile like peanut butter. According to Samara, adults should aim to get at least 1,000 mg of calcium per day (or more depending on their gender and age). It's so versatile, add it to shakes, sauces, drizzle on salads, and add it to hummus for an added boost of calcium. It is rich in vitamin B6 which helps with brain health. Learn more about other foods that aid in brain health in the Q & A section with Samara at the end of this book.

Organic Basil Seeds by Zen Basil are high in fiber. Just 2 tablespoons of Zen Basil Seeds offer 15 grams of fiber. Sprinkle them onto yogurt and add to shakes for a fiber boost. According to Samara, on average, men should aim for 30 grams of fiber per day and women should aim for 21 grams of fiber per day.

STRAWBERRY-CACAO SHAKE

MAKES 2 SHAKES

INGREDIENTS:

- 5 large frozen organic strawberries (or ¼ cup frozen organic cherries)
- 1 teaspoon cacao powder (or cocoa powder)
- 1 ½ cups nonfat milk (or milk alternative, almond, or oat milk)
- 1 teaspoon vanilla extract
- 1 teaspoon (or more) ground flaxseed
- 1 medjool date, pitted
- 1 tablespoon sugar-free maple syrup
- 1 tablespoon unflavored collagen powder (or chocolate protein powder)
- 2 medium-sized mason jars
- Straws for sipping
- High-speed blender

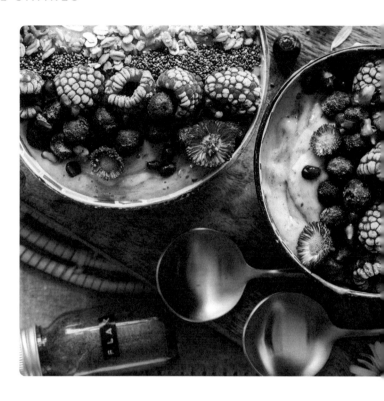

Mix all ingredients in the blender until creamy. If it's too thick add more milk. If it's too runny, add more ice.

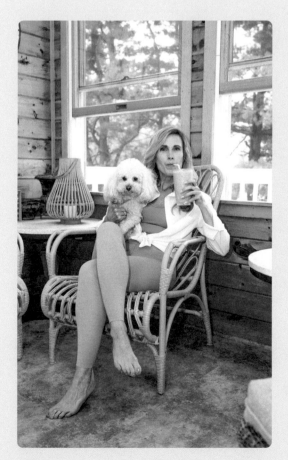

I start every day with a workout, sometimes getting up as early as 5:30 AM to get it done. My philosophy is that consistency is key. I've been doing this for over 30 years. You don't have to crush every workout, but you do have to remain consistent. My workouts include a combination of walking, jogging, the stationary bike, Pilates, yoga, stretching, toning, and weights. I also enjoy hitting the speed bag. My workouts set the tone for the rest of my day and allow me to be more productive. While I walk, I will often develop my recipes.

My early morning walks are all encompassing taking in nature's beauty and literally (and figuratively) grounding myself. I love watching the sun as it rises in the sky, setting the sky ablaze with hues of orange and red. I breathe in the crisp air, listen to the birds chirping and bees buzzing, and see my favorite horse in the distance. I remain in awe of my surroundings. It's a metaphor for life: I never walk alone.

After every early morning workout, I enjoy a shake that includes a healthy dose of fruit, sometimes spinach, a protein powder or collagen powder (which has added protein), and nonfat milk fortified with calcium or a milk alternative like almond milk. In the summer, I switch my shakes up and make them thicker, so I can have a smoothie bowl. I love adding frozen berries, kiwi which is high in fiber, and a little homemade granola to my smoothie bowls. Try these shake combos to start your day. They are delicious!

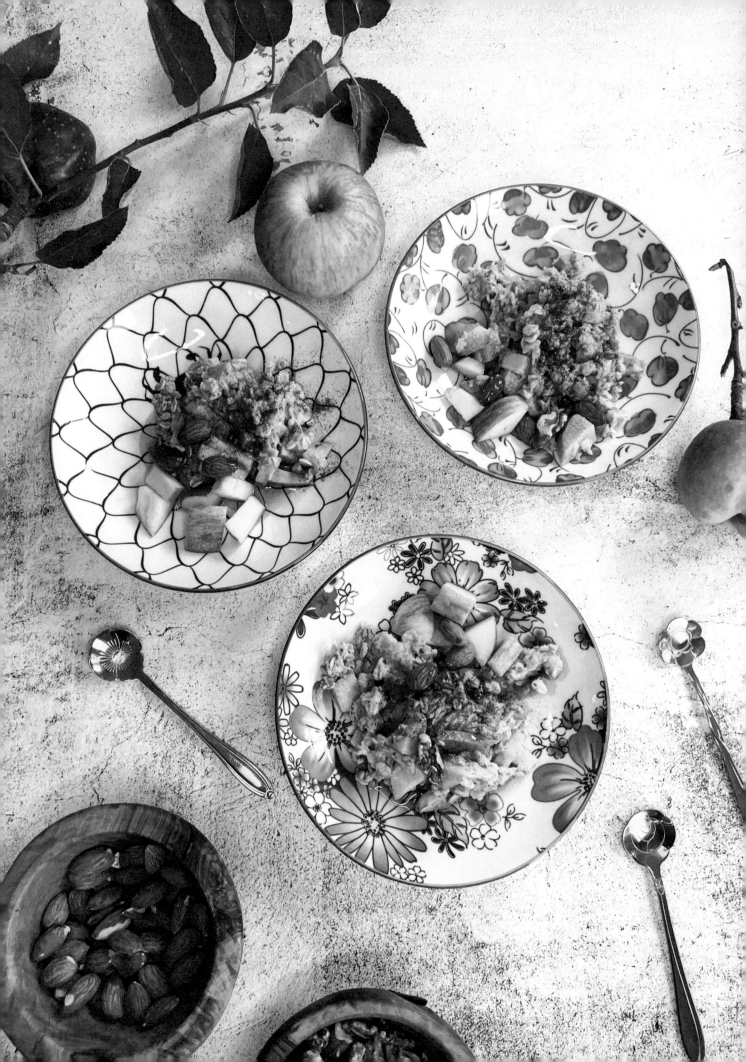

BAKED OATMEAL WITH APPLES
(Gluten Free)

SERVES 6–8

INGREDIENTS:

- 3 organic Fiji or Gala apples, peeled and finely diced, about 2 ½ cups
- 2 teaspoons granulated sugar
- 2 cups gluten-free rolled oats
- 1 ½ teaspoons baking powder
- 2 teaspoons cinnamon
- ½ teaspoon cardamon
- 2 cups low-fat milk (or milk substitute)
- ½ cup unsweetened applesauce
- ⅓ cup sugar-free maple syrup
- 1 tablespoon olive oil
- 2 teaspoons vanilla extract
- 1 large egg
- Non-stick cooking spray
- Cast-iron skillet
- Medium-sized baking dish
- Topping: drizzle of maple syrup and chopped almonds

Topping:

- ½ cup gluten-free rolled oats, pulsed
- ¼ cup light brown sugar, packed
- Sprinkle cinnamon
- 3 tablespoons salted butter, diced
- High-speed blender

Sometimes around midmorning, I will eat oatmeal. It's become a part of my daily morning routine. I wanted a change from cooking oatmeal on the stovetop, and that's when I created this super-easy oatmeal bake. It's all the ingredients you need to maintain good nutrition in one delicious bite. You can even prepare this the night before. Add more milk in the morning and pop it in the oven to warm it up while you are getting ready for work or school.

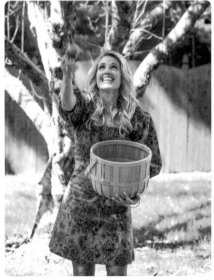
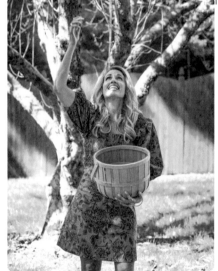
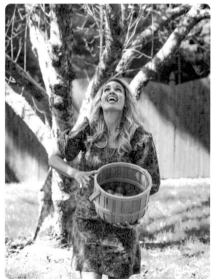
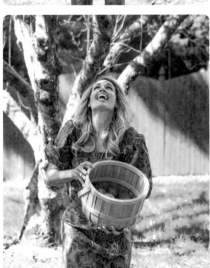
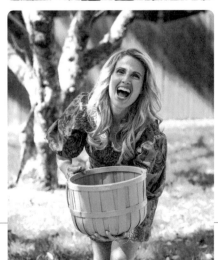
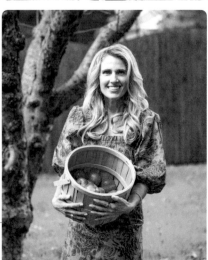

love to switch out the fruit depending on the season. In the fall, apples are great; I choose organic Fiji or Gala apples, which are so sweet. In the summer, I like fresh organic blueberries. It's an adaptable recipe, so choose any fruit in season. Top each bowl with maple syrup, which has hints of caramel and vanilla and pairs so well with the flavors in this dish. Add your favorite add-ins like chopped almonds or pecans. Delicious and nutritious! I eat this alongside protein-packed Greek yogurt to sustain my energy level.

Preheat the oven to 350 degrees. Grease the baking dish.

Peel the apples and finely dice into tiny bite-sized chunks. Add the apples to the skillet. Add a sprinkle of cinnamon and a little water so they steam. Cook the apples on medium heat for 15 minutes until caramelized and tender. You may add 1–2 teaspoons of sugar to further sweeten the apples. Add more water as needed so they don't dry out. Do not over saturate them.

In a large bowl, add the oats, baking powder, cinnamon, and cardamon, and mix.

In a separate bowl, add the milk, applesauce, maple syrup, oil, vanilla, and premixed egg, and whisk. Add the wet ingredients to the dry ingredients and mix. Allow it to sit while you continue to cook the apples.

Make the Topping.

Once apples are ready, prepare the topping. Pulse ½ cup of oats in the high-speed blender until you have achieved a powder-like consistency. Transfer the oat flour to a small bowl with brown sugar and a sprinkle of cinnamon. Combine the dry ingredients with a fork to get out any lumps. Next, in a microwave-safe bowl, melt the butter for 10 seconds and add it to the dry ingredients. Mix with your hands until you have achieved a crumbly texture.

Pour the oatmeal mixture into a greased dish. Add half of the apples to the top and press them into the mixture. Top with the topping and the remaining apples or you may just press all the apples into the oatmeal before adding topping.

Bake for 45–50 minutes in the middle of the oven. If you notice the bake browning too quickly, add foil and continue to bake covered. If you notice it's not cooking through, move to the top rack. Oven temperatures may vary.

Top each bowl with maple syrup, crushed nuts, and protein-rich Greek yogurt. Enjoy a lovely bowl of warm goodness. It's like a hug in a bowl.

This will keep for a few days covered tightly in the fridge. On day two it starts to taste more like bread pudding. I will soak a big spoonful in milk and reheat it in the microwave, this softens the bake. Then I drizzle on maple syrup. This is very reminiscent of bread pudding, something my dad loved so much.

Harvest tip: I developed this recipe to incorporate those juicy red apples in abundance in New Jersey from late August until October. Peak times for apple picking are from the beginning of September until October 15th. I am very lucky to have apple trees on my property. Some years they have big blooms.

Apple picking tip: Remember this tip when you go apple picking. One sign that apples are ready to be picked is when the color is deepening. Taste it to be sure it's ready! It should be sweet. A gentle twist and it should come right off, leaving a stem intact, otherwise if you have to tug at it, it's likely not ready, so pick another apple.

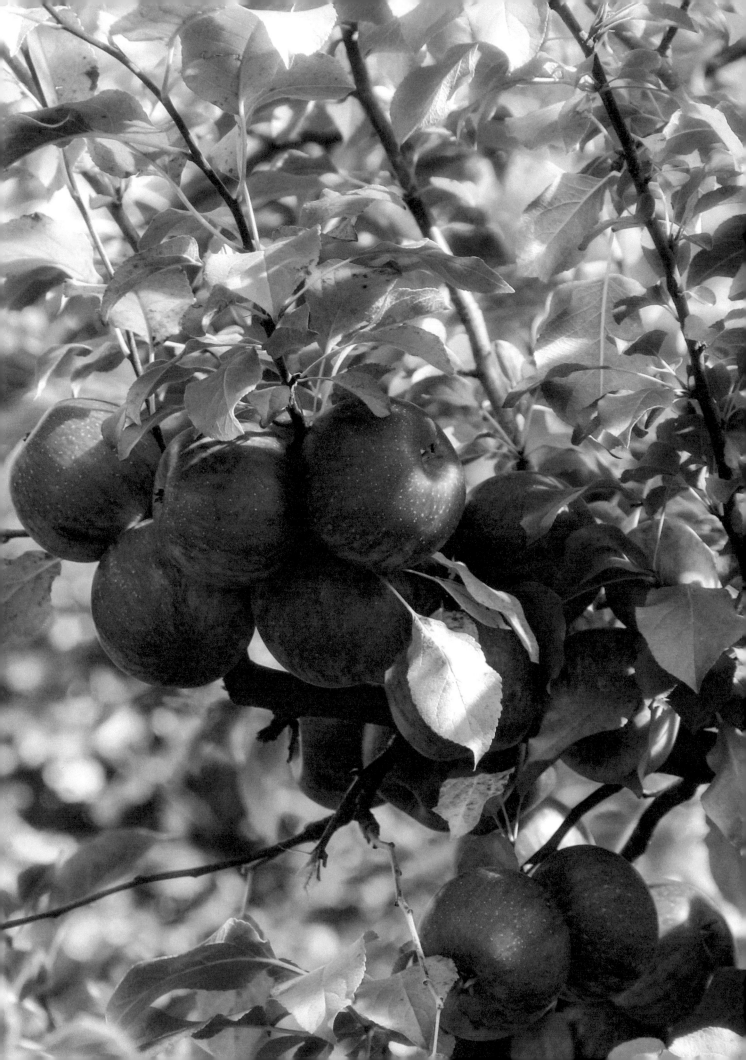

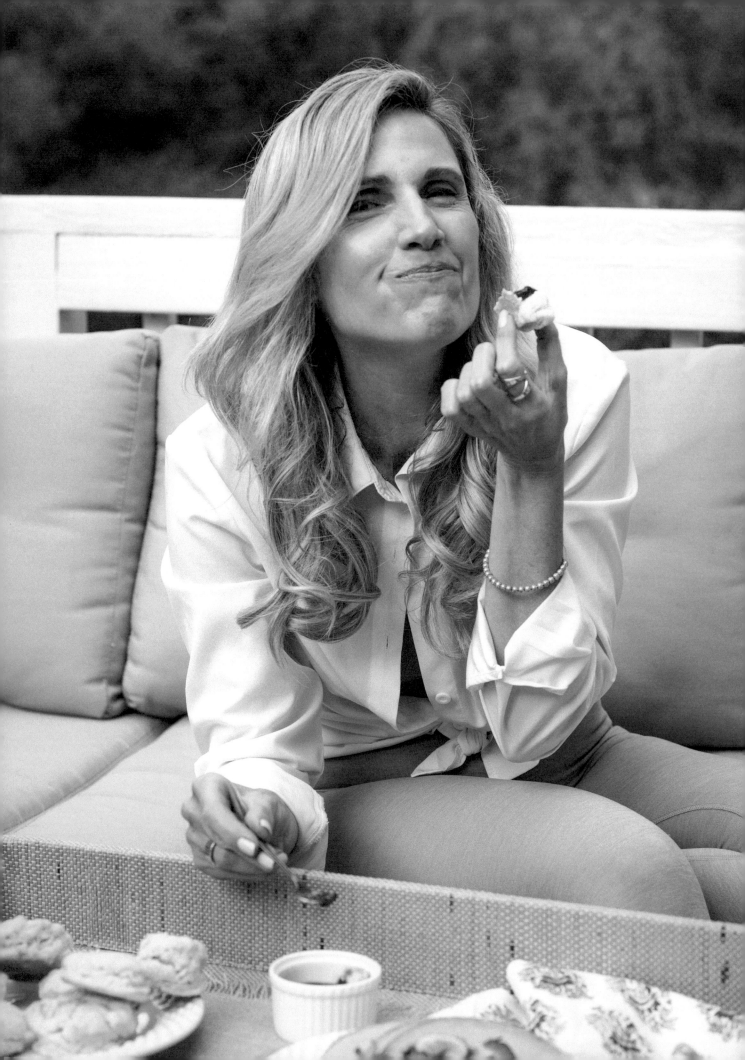

SAVORY MORNINGS

CHAI-SPICED PUMPKIN LOAF
(Gluten Free)

EVERYTHING BAGELS
(Gluten Free)

JAPANESE YAM LOAF
(Gluten Free)

FLAKY BISCUITS

LEMON POPPY SEED MUFFINS
(Gluten Free)

AREPAS
(Gluten Free)

CHAI-SPICED PUMPKIN LOAF
(Gluten Free)

Pumpkin pairs well with warming spices like ginger, cinnamon, and nutmeg, but the addition of lavender and rosemary really enhances the flavors in this cake. It's an unexpected pairing that will wow your guests. The Chai Spice Blend is great to keep on hand for other fall recipes. Be sure to plant lavender in your garden, so you can use it in recipes all year long.

INGREDIENTS:

- 1 cup gluten-free rolled oats, pulsed
- 1 cup super-fine almond flour, spooned and leveled
- 2 teaspoons Chai Spice Blend (recipe follows)
- ½ teaspoon dried culinary lavender flowers
- ½ tablespoon dried rosemary
- 1 cup pumpkin purée (store-bought), strained
- ¾ cup light brown sugar
- 1 cup olive oil
- 1 tablespoon molasses
- 2 teaspoons vanilla extract
- 1 large egg, room temperature
- 1 teaspoon baking soda
- ½ teaspoon baking powder
- ¾ teaspoon xanthan gum (optional)
- Loaf pan
- Stand mixer with paddle attachment
- High-speed blender
- Strainer
- Mortar and pestle
- Cheesecloth

Lavender Simple Syrup:

- ½ cup water
- ½ cup granulated sugar
- ½ teaspoon dried culinary lavender flowers

Chai Spice Blend:

- ½ teaspoon cinnamon
- ½ teaspoon ginger
- ½ teaspoon cardamom
- ½ teaspoon pumpkin pie spice
- ¼ teaspoon ground cloves (optional)

Topping:

- Dash of cinnamon, ginger, cardamom, and pumpkin pie spice
- 1 tablespoon light brown sugar
- 2–3 tablespoons salted butter, melted

Lavender Icing:

- ½ cup powdered sugar
- 2 tablespoons Lavender Simple Syrup (recipe follows)

Preheat the oven to 325 degrees. This is the preferred temperature for baking loaves.

Make the Lavender Simple Syrup.

In a small pot, stir together equal parts water and sugar. Bring to a boil, stir, and let the sugar dissolve. Stir until translucent. This creates the simple syrup, then you can infuse flavor. Take it off the burner, add in the lavender flowers and give it a quick stir, and cover. Let it steep until it's cool, strain, and discard flowers. Then refrigerate until ready to use. Use this to infuse flavor into cocktails, cakes, or cookies. Store in an air-tight container in the refrigerator for 1–2 weeks. You can use other garden herbs like thyme, rosemary, or mint too.

> Use fragrant English lavender. This is culinary lavender and is available at farmer's markets, or online. I harvest the lavender from my garden in the summer, dry it, and jar it for use during the year and for this delicious loaf. Alternatively, you can buy lavender simple syrup.

Fun fact: Using fresh pumpkin in this recipe is another healthy alternative. Jack once planted an entire pumpkin in the ground, and we grew a very large, ever-growing pumpkin patch. It was something to see. True story. Ha-ha!

In the high-speed blender, add the oats and pulse about 2 minutes to create a powder-like consistency. Some tiny bits will remain. Stir to redistribute oats. Add the almond flour and pulse for 1 minute.

Over a large bowl, pour the combined flour mixture into a strainer a little at a time. With the back of a spoon stir the mixture to break up the clumps. Some of the mixture will not go through a very fine strainer, which is fine. We just want to break up the clumps. Set the flour mixture aside.

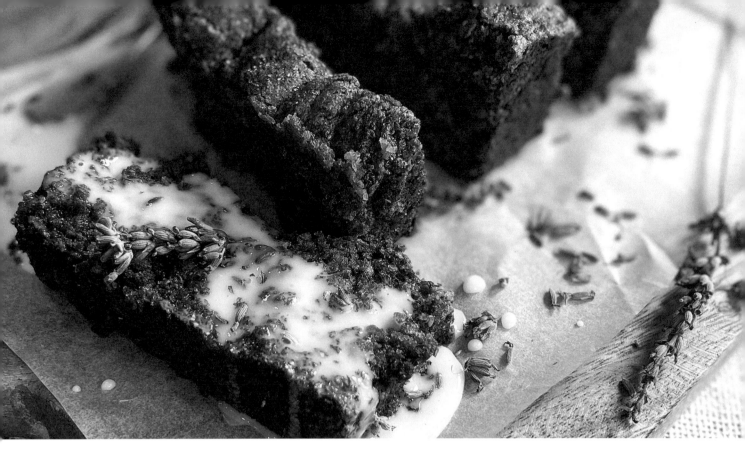

Make the Chai Spice Blend.

This is so fragrant. Make a big batch and store it in a jar. Use it in cakes & cookies all year long.

In a small bowl, add the cinnamon, ginger, cardamom, and pumpkin pie spice and mix. In a mortar and pestle, add the rosemary and lavender and break it up. Mix with chai spices. Set this aside.

Add the pumpkin purée into a cheesecloth and gently strain out the excess liquid over the sink.

In the bowl of the stand mixer, add the strained pumpkin purée, sugar, olive oil, molasses, and vanilla. Mix on medium speed. Last, add the premixed egg and mix on medium speed until combined.

Add the baking soda, baking powder, xanthan gum, chai spices (including lavender and rosemary) and whisk with the flour mixture. Combine the dry ingredients with the wet ingredients and mix for 1 minute on medium speed, scraping down the sides and bottom of the bowl.

Prepare the loaf pan with parchment paper. Pour the mixture in the loaf pan.

Prepare the Topping.

Add the spices and sugar and mix. Pour the butter over the loaf. You may not need all of it. Sprinkle on the spices/ sugar mixture.

Bake on the top shelf for about 1 hour and 15 minutes. It's best to bake at 325 degrees and go longer, so it doesn't burn at a higher temperature and remain soggy on the inside.

Allow it to cool for about 20 minutes in the loaf pan. Then pick up the ends of the parchment paper and lift the loaf onto a cooling rack. This is the hardest part of the recipe because this is the most fragrant cake and it's hard to resist eating it before it's ready because it smells so good.

Cool the loaf an additional hour before you cut into it. It's so delicate that cutting slices may be a little challenging, so the longer you let it sit–even overnight–the better. I made this recipe multiple times without the xanthan gum and it was great, but the xanthan gum will hold it together nicely so you can cut perfect slices.

Loaf cutting tip: turn the loaf on its side, then cut the individual slices. This will keep the top of the cake intact.

Prepare the Lavender Icing.

Mix the powdered sugar with the lavender syrup and whisk. Pour on each slice.

This recipe was featured in The Art of Celebrating Magazine by Akeshi Akinseye Holiday 2022 Issue. I was honored to be featured and have my work highlighted.

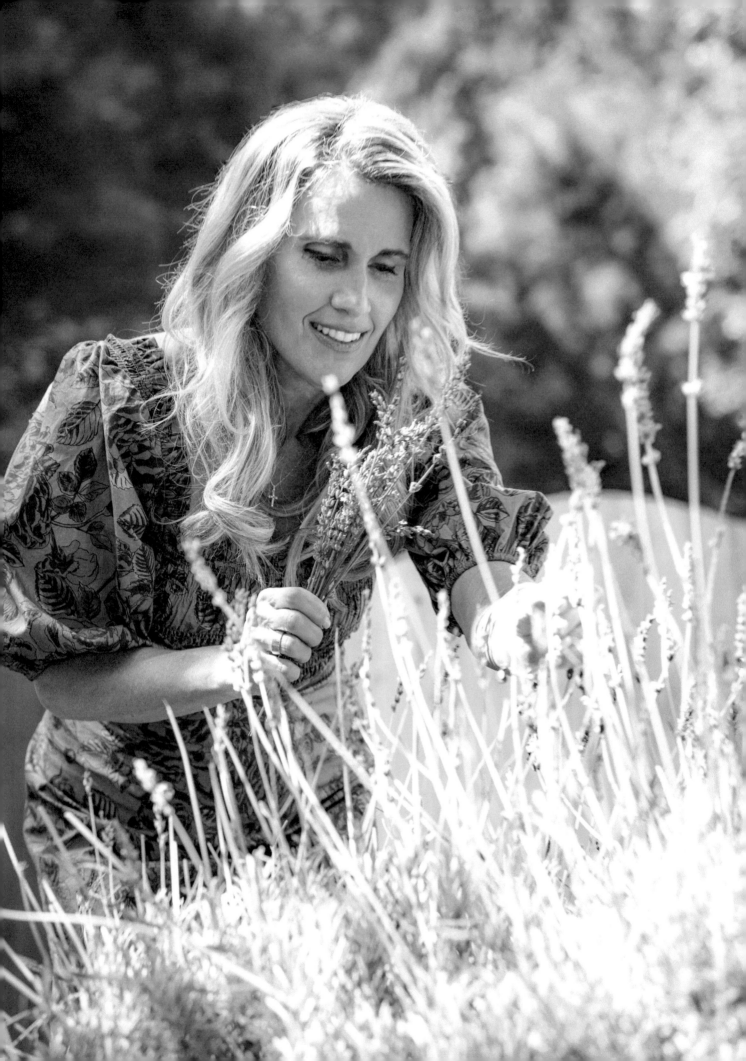

LAVENDER IN THE BREEZE

A strong gust of wind blows the aromatic scent
I can smell the lavender wafting in the breezy air
Recalling the fragrant cakes and cookies made all year
The lavender cut into tidy bunches, dried in the sweltering sun
Kept in tiny glass jars
Harvest has come   I can smell it in the air
The days are longer, and the sun grows hot against my flushed face
It's time for harvest
I run to my lavender fields eager to see the tall spiky flowers
The bees are buzzing and collecting the nectar
I must be quick and not disturb them
In one fell swoop, I gather and cut the flowers
And place them in my gardener's basket
As I walk inside
I stand still for a moment, holding the lavender close to my face
The pungent scent permeates through my nose
I can almost taste the cake I'll make with it.
Harvest has come

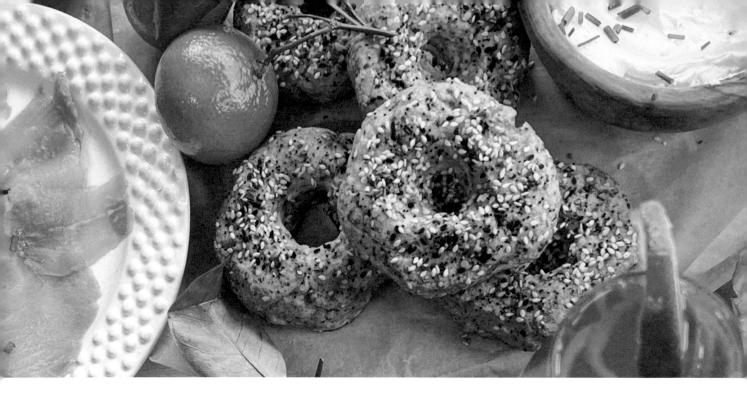

EVERYTHING BAGELS
(Gluten Free)

I worked tirelessly creating this bagel recipe for those of you who are living a gluten-free lifestyle. I know finding a good gluten-free bagel can be a challenge. This recipe is part creative and part scientific experimentation, the outcome being nothing less than delicious. The taste is like nothing else you've ever tasted.

INGREDIENTS:

- 2 ¼ teaspoons quick-rise yeast, dissolved in ¼ cup warm water
- ½ tablespoon granulated sugar
- 1 ¼ cup white rice flour (or brown rice flour), spooned and leveled
- 1 ¼ cup tapioca flour, spooned and leveled
- 1 ¼ cup super-fine almond flour, spooned and leveled
- 4 tablespoons flax meal
- 1 teaspoon baking soda
- ¾ teaspoon xanthan gum
- ½ teaspoon cream of tartar
- 2 teaspoons table or sea salt
- ¾ cup warm water, drizzle in while mixer is on until dough forms
- Stand mixer with hook attachment
- Slotted spoon
- Large, wide-mouthed pot
- Pastry cutter
- Wood pastry board
- Pastry brush

Other ingredients:

- Olive oil
- 1 tablespoon honey
- 1 large baking sheet with parchment paper
- 1 large egg, premixed
- Everything bagel seasonings, poppy seeds, or sesame seeds

Note: Rapid-rise or quick-rise yeast work great for these bagels, but active dry yeast is equally good. It may take longer for the dough to double.

Preheat the oven to 350 degrees. I like to start with a warm oven, so I have a warm place for my bagels/bread to rise on the stovetop. After 30 minutes you can turn off the oven. The bagels bake at a much higher temperature.

First, dissolve the yeast in ¼ cup warm water and stir with a fork. Transfer the yeast mixture to the stand mixer bowl. Add the sugar and stir again. Let this sit 5–10 minutes.

In another bowl, add the flours, flax meal, baking soda, xanthan gum, cream of tartar, and salt. Whisk until well combined.

Note: It is a good idea to whisk the almond flour separately to break up the chunks, then measure for this recipe.

Add the dry ingredients to the wet ingredients in the stand mixer bowl, and slowly drizzle in the water. If it's still a little wet, add 1 tablespoon of rice flour at a time. If it's a little dry, add 1 tablespoon of water at a time. This is a good rule of thumb for bread too. It may be dry if you did not precisely measure your ingredients.

Once the dough has formed together and pulls away from the sides of the bowl, dump it onto a lightly floured wood board or clean work surface. Add a little olive oil to the bowl, dump the dough back in, and cover the bowl. Let it sit on the stovetop, or in a warm spot in your home, for 1–1 ½ hours.

Preheat the oven to 425 degrees.

Once the dough doubles in size, cut 6 equal-sized pieces using a pastry cutter. Shape each piece into a ball of dough. If you prefer a bigger bagel, make 4 equal-sized pieces.

Press a hole through the center of the ball and gently stretch out the center. You want to be sure you have a nicely rounded hole in the center, so you get that quintessential bagel shape. Cover the bagels for 15 minutes. Keep them on the stovetop where it's warm, so they puff up.

In the meantime, prepare the water bath. Bring a huge pot of water to a rapid boil. Be sure to add in 1 tablespoon or more of honey, this will brown the bagels once baked. Turn down the heat a little and drop in 3 bagels at a time using a slotted spoon.

Important: They should float to the surface, then start counting for 1 minute.

Flip the bagels after 1 minute and count an additional minute, or up to 2 minutes. Then flip back to the front side and transfer to the parchment-lined baking sheet. Be sure to drain the bagel over the pot of water, so the parchment paper does not get soggy. If it does, dry it with a paper towel.

Brush the bagels with the egg wash and add the seasonings of your choice. This is especially helpful because if you have any cracks the egg wash will fill them in.

Bake for 30–33 minutes (or longer, if you made them bigger) until golden brown, turning the pan halfway through.

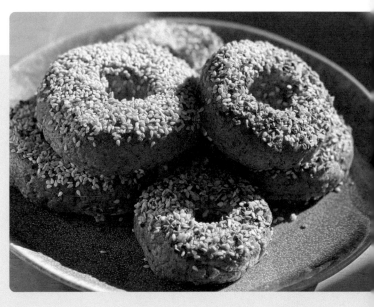

The science behind the bagel. First, let's delve into the science behind bread made with flour like all-purpose flour. The yeast, once activated in your recipe, will create and release carbon dioxide. The gluten acts as a net, encapsulating the air bubbles and maintaining the airy structure of the bagel or bread once baked.

In the case of a gluten-free bagel, we cannot rely upon gluten as a net, so to speak. Instead, we use the yeast, which still produces the bubbles along with the baking powder (a leavening agent), and cream of tartar (an acid), which will further activate this process. The xanthan gum, however, will serve to hold the structure of the bagel, trapping that air inside the dough, allowing it to rise, and maintaining the structure of the bread.

In this recipe especially, the xanthan gum does a great job creating some elasticity and yielding a chewy bagel. It produces a nice texture that cannot be achieved in baking without it.

To knead or not to knead? That is the question.

While wheat breads require kneading to develop the gluten proteins into an elastic dough, gluten-free bread dough gets its consistency from xanthan gum added to the flour. This means kneading isn't required and a mix to just incorporate ingredients is sufficient.

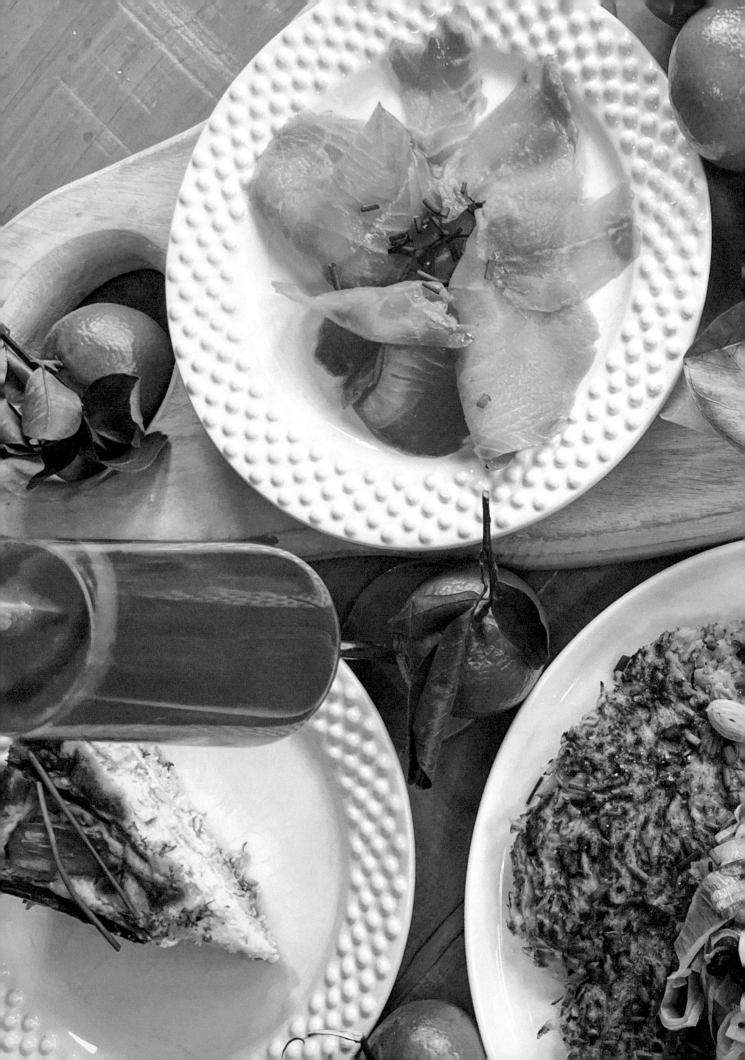

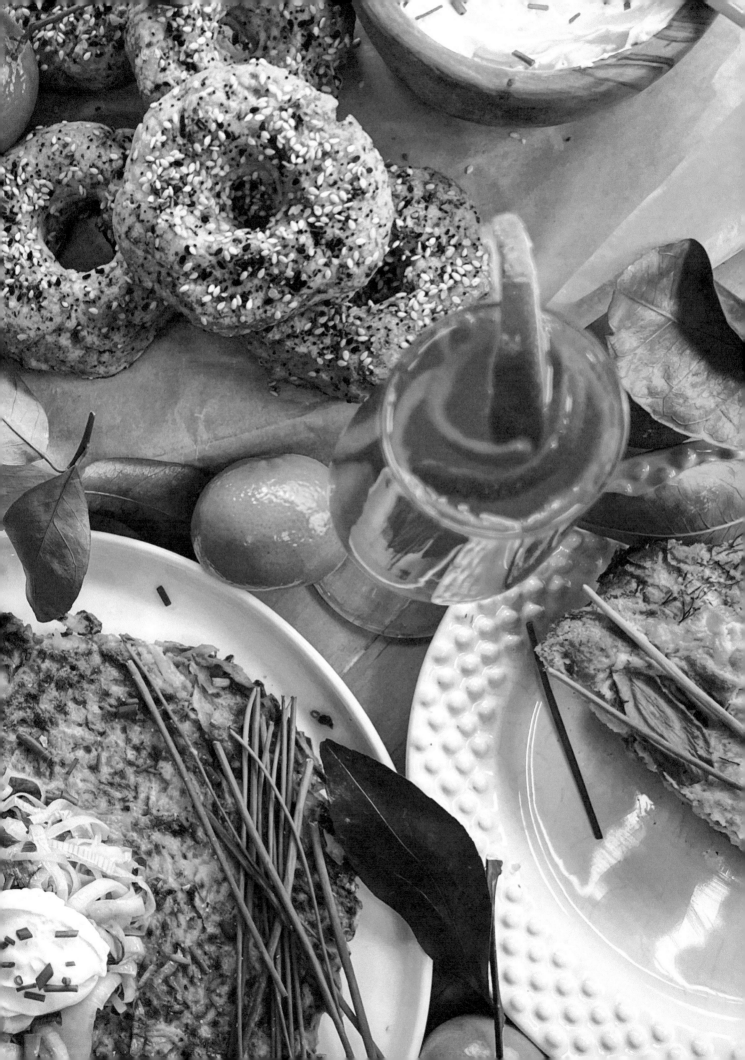

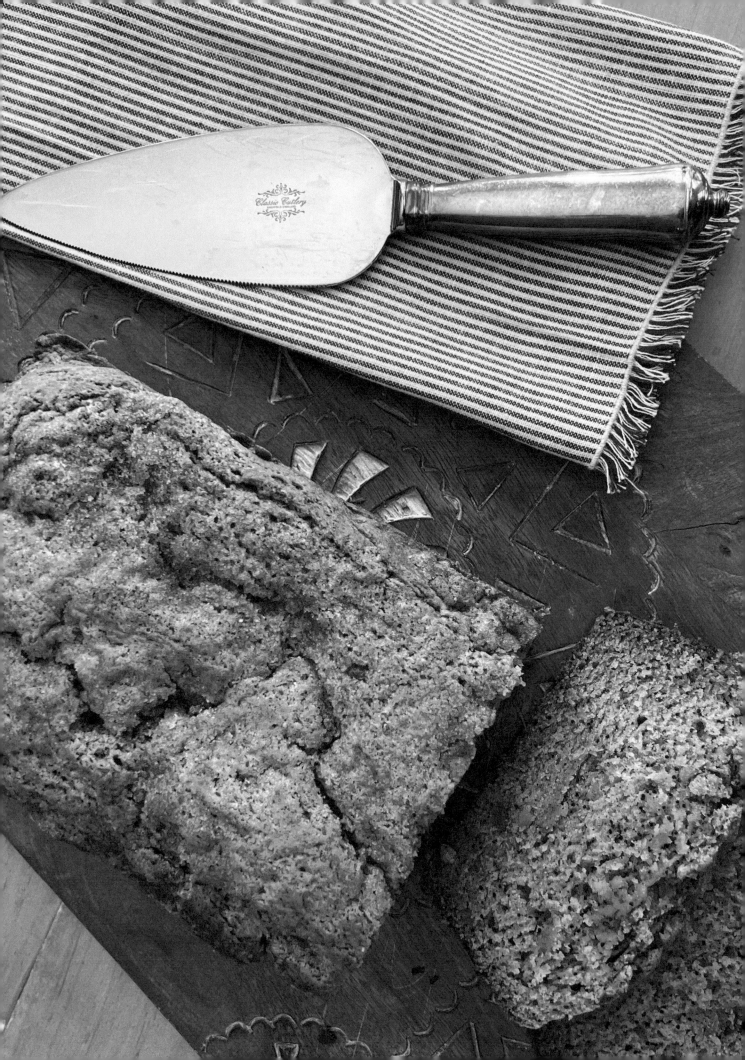

JAPANESE SWEET POTATO LOAF
(Gluten Free)

Japanese sweet potatoes have purple skin and a sweet, nutty flavor which make a winning combination in this bread recipe. Japanese sweet potato has a slightly dry, white flesh that's rich in fiber and vitamin C.

INGREDIENTS:

- 1 cup mashed organic Japanese Sweet Potato (about 1 large potato)
- ½ cup granulated sugar
- ¼ cup light brown sugar
- ¾ cup extra virgin olive oil
- 1 teaspoon vanilla extract
- 2 tablespoons tahini
- 2 tablespoons light sour cream
- ⅓ cup nonfat milk plus 3–4 tablespoons to loosen batter
- 2 tablespoons poppy seeds
- 1 egg
- 1 ¾ cup gluten-free flour (I used King Arthur Baking Company's Gluten-Free Measure for Measure Flour), spooned and leveled
- 1 teaspoon baking powder
- 1 teaspoon baking soda
- 1 teaspoon cinnamon
- 1 teaspoon ground ginger
- Non-stick cooking spray
- Loaf pan
- Stand mixer with paddle attachment

Topping:

- ¼ cup light brown sugar
- ½ teaspoon ginger
- 3 tablespoons salted butter, melted

Mascarpone-Honey Lemon Spread Ingredients:

- 4 tablespoons mascarpone cheese, room temperature
- ½ small lemon, squeezed (about ½ tablespoon)
- ½ teaspoon clear vanilla extract
- 1–2 tablespoons organic honey

In the stand mixer bowl, add the cooked and peeled sweet potato. Mix on medium speed to get out any lumps. This is an important step. You may also mash it first and then add it to the stand mixer. Next, add the sugars, olive oil, vanilla, tahini, sour cream, and milk. Mix on medium speed until well combined and no lumps remain.

In a medium-sized bowl, add the flour, baking powder, baking soda, cinnamon, ginger, and poppy seeds. Whisk until well combined.

Note: Be sure the gluten-free flour you are using includes xanthan gum in the ingredient listing; if it doesn't, add ½ teaspoon to this cake. Alternatively, swap out the gluten-free flour for cake flour.

Add the dry ingredients to the stand mixer bowl with the wet ingredients. Mix on medium speed until the batter is smooth.

Spray the loaf pan with non-stick cook spray or line it with parchment paper.

Prepare the Topping.

In a small bowl, combine the sugar, ginger, and melted butter. Mix to combine and add to the top of the bread right before baking.

Bake at 350 for 50–55 minutes. Continue to bake until springy and a toothpick comes out clean. Allow cake to cool for about 20 minutes in the loaf pan, and then carefully transfer the cake to a cooling rack to continue to cool.

Prepare the Mascarpone-Honey Lemon Spread.

Combine the room temperature cheese with the lemon juice, vanilla, and honey. Mix to combine. If you are serving the cake right away, you may leave it at room temperature, otherwise it should be refrigerated.

For my baking recipes, feel free to adjust the sugar. You may try a sugar substitute as well or just use less sugar in the recipe if you prefer.

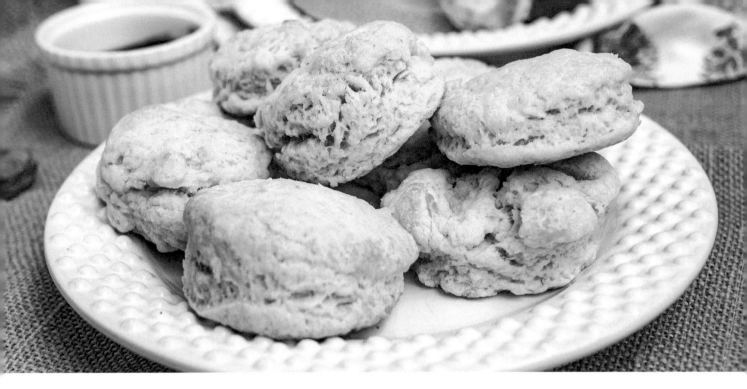

FLAKY BISCUITS

MAKES 14-15 BISCUITS

INGREDIENTS:

- 3 cups all-purpose flour (or gluten-free flour)
- 1 tablespoon baking powder
- 1 tablespoon granulated sugar
- 1 teaspoon table salt
- 1 cup milk (whole, 2%, low-fat, or buttermilk)
- 6 tablespoons salted butter, cold and finely grated
- 2 ¾-inch biscuit cutter (or glass with 2 ¾-inch opening)
- ½ stick salted butter, melted
- Excess flour for dusting
- Box grater
- Pastry brush
- Wood pastry board

Preheat the oven to 425 degrees.

In a large bowl, add the flour, baking powder, sugar, and salt, and whisk. Next, add the milk and grated butter. Mix with clean hands to fully combine. Dumping it onto a clean, lightly floured work surface will make this easier. If it's sticky, add 1 tablespoon of flour at a time, until it is no longer sticky.

Once the butter is fully incorporated and you have formed a cohesive dough, shape it into a rectangle. Then fold dough in half, press the layers together, and turn. Keep folding, pressing, and turning. This creates the flaky layers. Do this about 5 times.

Using your hands, press the dough flat into about 1-inch thickness. Dip the biscuit cutter or glass in flour and cut into biscuits. Reshape any excess, press it down, and make another biscuit until all the dough is used.

Place the biscuits onto a parchment-lined baking sheet. Brush the tops and sides with melted butter. Bake in the oven for about 12 minutes until the tops are golden.

These are so delicious and are best fresh from the oven. Serve with a homemade jam made from fresh fruit like raspberries, strawberreis, or figs, and a healthy serving of fruit to make this a well-balanced breakfast.

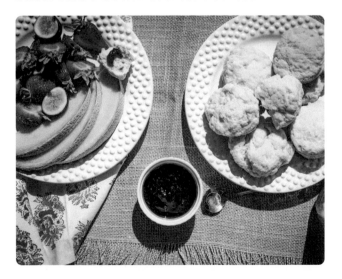

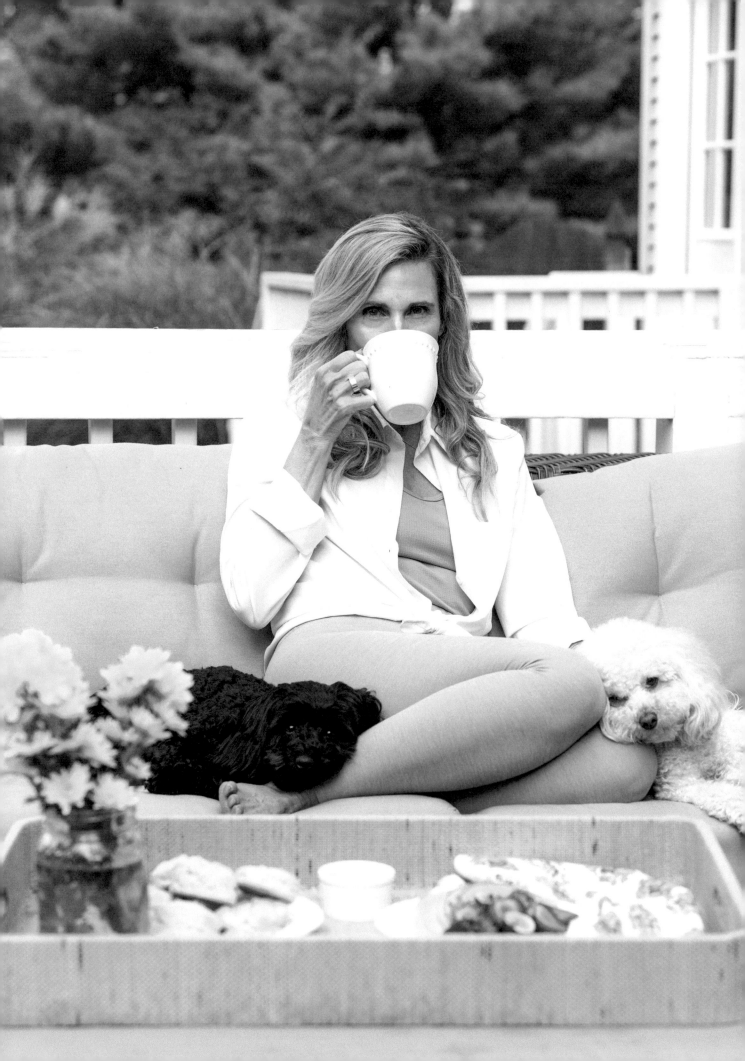

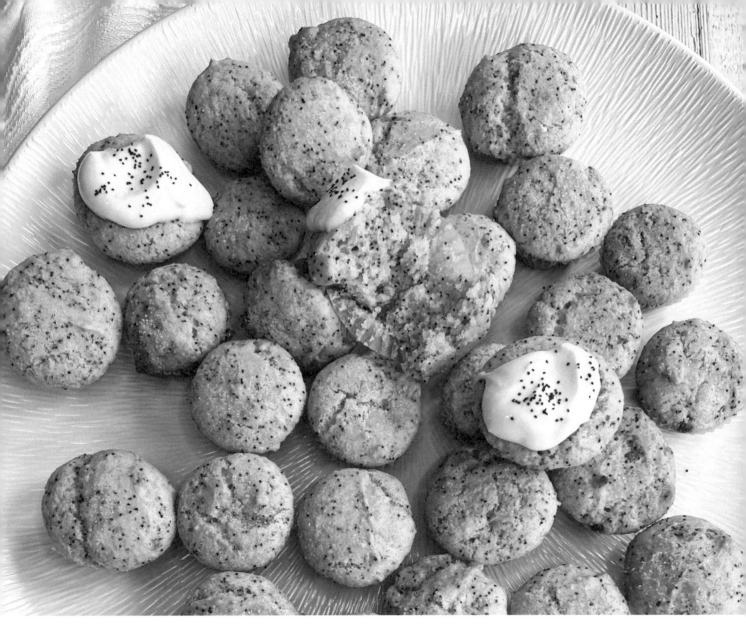

LEMON POPPY SEED MUFFINS
(Gluten Free)

These muffins are bursting with citrus flavor, but they lean toward savory with the addition of poppy seeds and almond flour. They are a great addition to any brunch or tea. And although a fair amount of experimentation was involved in this recipe, I am happy to say that the outcome is nothing less than delicious. I have experimented with using only almond flour and the muffins were very gummy, so I prefer using a blend of flours. I like King Arthur Baking Company's Gluten-Free Measure for Measure Flour combined with super-fine almond flour for a winning combination. If your flour doesn't contain xanthan gum, add ½ teaspoon to this recipe. Xanthan gum will help hold the muffins together. Alternatively, using all-purpose flour and almond flour is equally good if you are not gluten-free.

The Creamy Yogurt-Lemon Icing is super light and lemony. It's so good without being overly sweet like most icings. With that said, if you want to make these muffins sweeter, more like a cupcake, you can use butter cream icing and top with more poppy seeds.

INGREDIENTS:

- ¼ cup light brown sugar, packed
- ½ cup granulated sugar, plus more for topping
- ¾ cup extra virgin olive oil (or vegetable oil)
- 2 tablespoons light cream cheese, room temperature
- 2 tablespoons light sour cream, room temperature
- 1 lemon, squeezed (3 tablespoons or more)
- 1 lemon, zested
- 2 large eggs, room temperature
- 1 ¼ cups gluten-free flour (or all-purpose flour), spooned and leveled
- 1 cup super-fine almond flour, spooned and leveled
- ½ teaspoon baking soda
- 1 teaspoon baking powder
- 2 tablespoons poppy seeds, plus more for topping
- Stand mixer with paddle attachment
- Mini-muffin tin, 24 muffins
- Mini-muffin tin liners
- Whisk

Creamy Yogurt-Lemon Icing:

- ¾ –1 cup plain Greek yogurt (2%, or nonfat)
- 1 tablespoon light cream cheese, room temperature
- 1 tablespoon light sour cream
- 1 teaspoon lemon juice, freshly squeezed
- 3 tablespoons of powdered sugar

Preheat the oven to 350 degrees.

In the stand mixer bowl with paddle attachment, add the brown sugar. Mix on low to break up any lumps, or you can do this with a fork prior to adding it to the mixer. Then add the granulated sugar, olive oil (or vegetable oil), cream cheese, and sour cream. Mix on medium speed until it forms a yellow batter. Next, add the lemon juice and zest. Mix on medium speed. While the mixer is still on, stream in the premixed eggs. Mix on medium speed for 30 seconds just to incorporate the eggs, do not over mix.

> *Baker's tip: To flavor the sugar, zest the lemon into the sugar and mix with your hands to infuse lemon flavor. For the best taste, choose organic lemons for this recipe. Be sure to wash them before zesting. This applies to all my recipes requiring fruit. Organic fruit is always a good choice to avoid unnecessary pesticides.*

In a large bowl, add the flour, baking soda, and baking powder. Whisk to break up any lumps. Then add the poppy seeds and whisk to combine.

Add the flour mixture into the stand mixer bowl along with the other ingredients. Mix until all the ingredients are well combined. Use a spatula to fully incorporate ingredients that may be stuck on the bottom and sides of the bowl.

Line the muffin tins with the paper liners and add 1 heaping tablespoon (or slightly more) of batter. Add a pinch of sugar to the top of each muffin.

Bake for about 20 minutes until springy and golden. If you notice they aren't browning (this will happen if you didn't add the sugar on top) crank the heat up to 375 degrees for the last minute or 2.

Make the Creamy Yogurt-Lemon Icing:

In a bowl, add all the ingredients and whisk until fluffy. Place in the fridge until you are ready to use. Add a dollop to cooled cupcakes. Top with more poppy seeds or lemon zest.

Once the cupcakes are done, place them onto a cooling rack to cool for 15 minutes. Ice and enjoy!

Any leftover icing should be refrigerated.

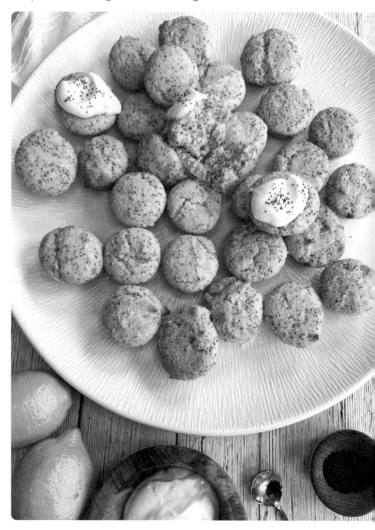

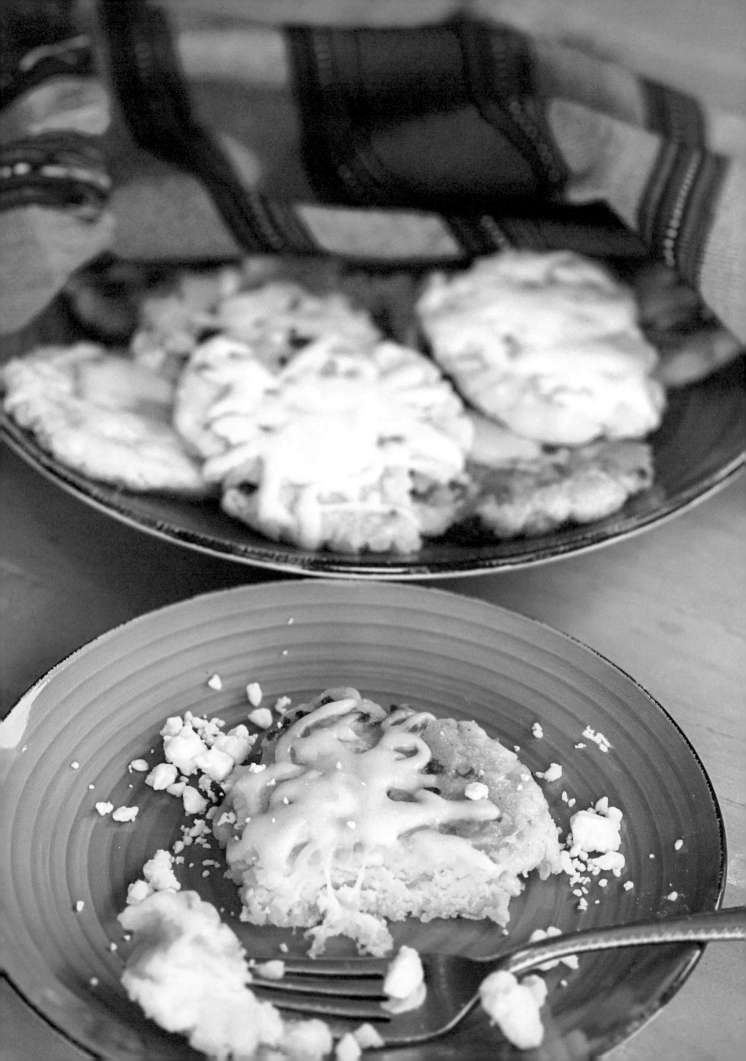

AREPAS
(Gluten Free)

INGREDIENTS:

- 1 cup white sweet corn, frozen (or cooked fresh corn)
- 2 cups masarepa yellow corn meal (pre-cooked)
- ½– ¾ cup shredded low-fat mozzarella cheese
- Water as needed (about 1 ¾ cups)
- Salt to taste
- Salted butter
- Extra virgin olive oil
- Medium-sized frying pan
- High-speed blender

Arepas are flat, round, unleavened patties of soaked, ground kernels of maize (or corn as we know it). Nowadays pre-cooked and finely ground corn meal is used more frequently.

Arepas may be grilled, baked, fried, boiled, or steamed. The characteristics vary by color, flavor, size, and the food with which it may be stuffed or topped. Some arepas are filled with butter or cheese and then baked. Fried arepas are often eaten in northern South American countries like Columbia and Venezuela, where they are filled and topped with white cheese. Some cheese choices are mozzarella or queso fresco for topping. They are popular for breakfast, lunch, or even dinner.

Isabel, Maggie's friend, introduced us to arepas. She does not add the blended corn to her Columbian version. My version of arepas, I add in a little ground sweet white corn for added texture and taste. Adding lots of mozzarella cheese and butter is a must. Add water as needed to properly form the arepas. Isabel brought back this beautiful towel from Columbia for me to use when I make my arepas. It keeps the arepas warm.

Choosing the right flour is *essential* to mastering this recipe. Always look for the note "perfect for arepas" on the package of masarepa yellow corn meal which is pre-cooked and finely ground. If it's not properly ground corn meal, the arepas will taste very gritty and be inedible.

Cook the frozen corn according to package directions. Alternatively, use fresh cooked corn. Next, add the cooked corn to the blender. Mix until chunky. Add the corn mixture to the bowl, along with the corn meal and mozzarella cheese and mix. Add a little water at a time to create a dough that holds together once squeezed, similar to a playdough consistency. Add a little salt to the mixture. You will top each arepa with salt, so don't add too much.

Make 10 Arepas:

Add 3–4 arepas at at time to an oiled skillet. Add a lid to encapsulate the heat. Heat for 4 minutes a side, pressing down the arepa with a spatula. Flip and continue to heat without the lid for 4 additional minutes.

Top each arepa with salt, butter, and then more mozzarella cheese. You can put the lid over them for 30 seconds to melt the cheese.

Serve on a plate with some corn and quesa fresco or cotija cheese. These are absolutely delicious!

Trouble shooting some possible concerns:

- *The dough looks a little dry in spots. Add 1 tablespoon at a time of water and keep squeezing the dough to form it together. Don't let it get too wet.*

- *The arepas are not getting golden brown. The heat should be between medium and medium-high.*

- *The arepas are still uncooked in the center. Be sure to press them down and slighly flatten so they cook through.*

- *The arepas are sticking to the pan. Choose a non-stick frying pan and add oil (about 3–4 tablespoons each time you cook 4 arepas).*

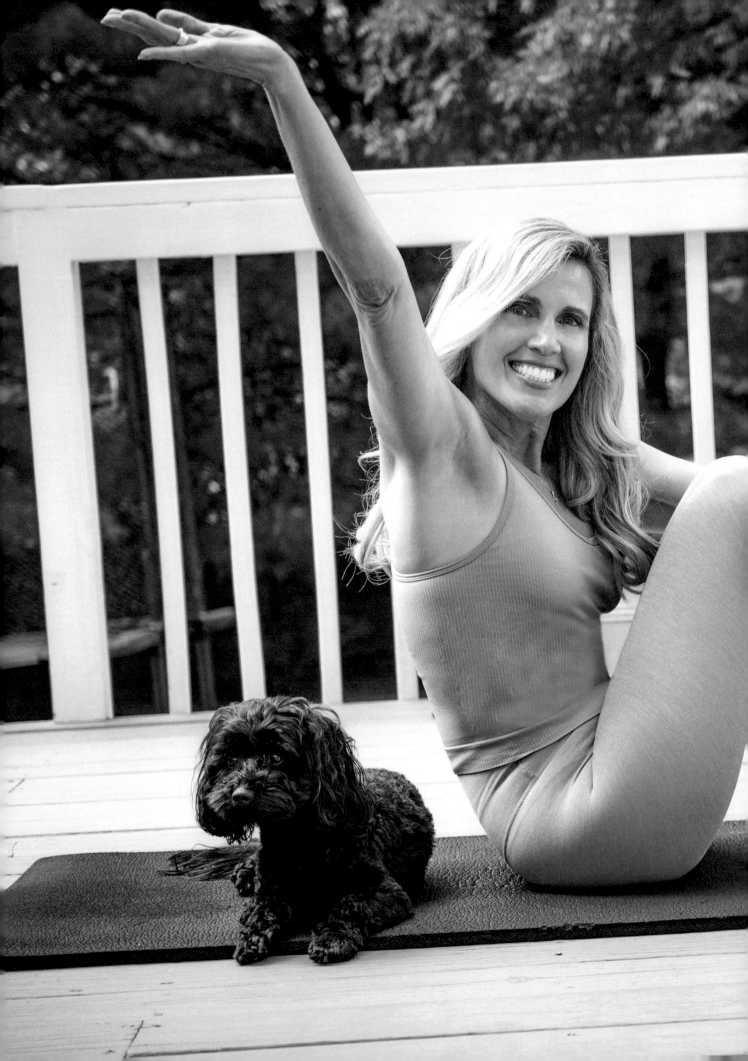

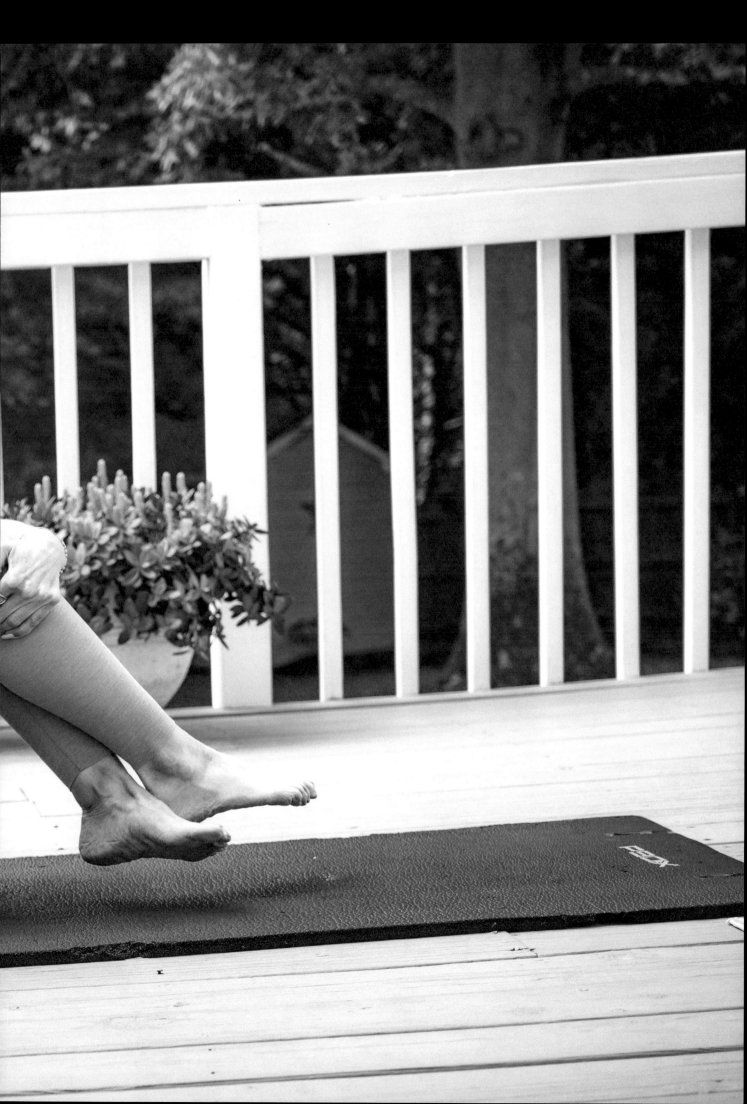

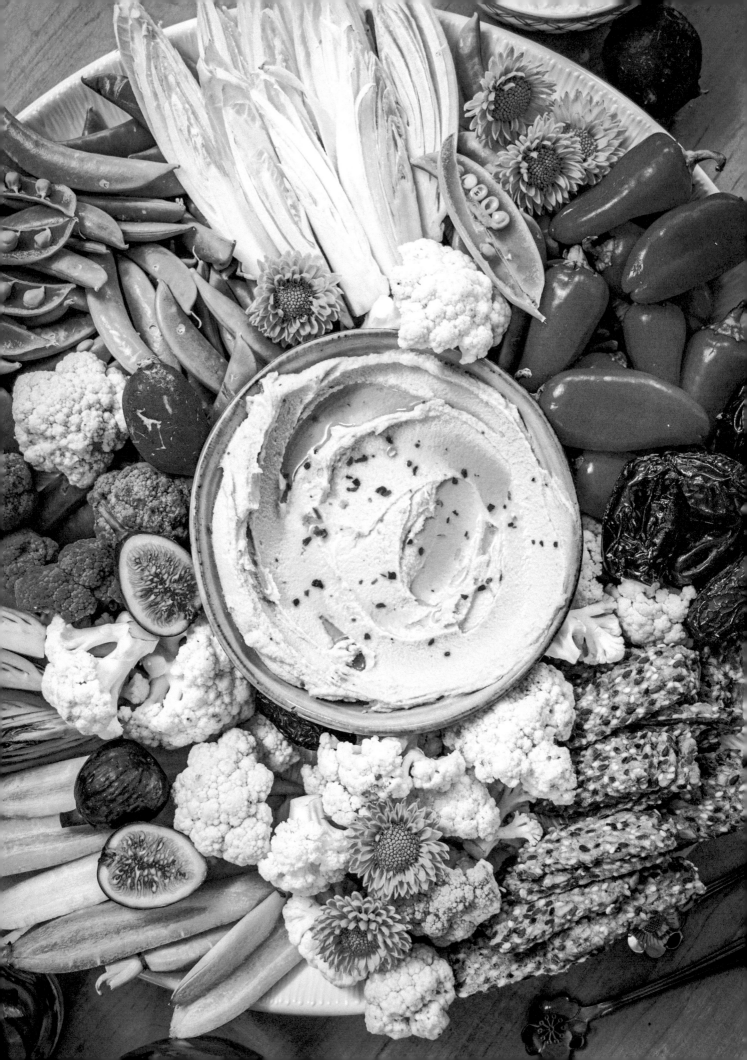

APPETIZERS
AND STARTERS

MEZZE PLATTER

JALAPEÑO POPPERS
(Gluten Free)

QUINOA AND BLACK BEAN BAKE
(Gluten Free)

MINI GOAT CHEESE AND PROSCIUTTO PIZZAS

MINI TURKEY MEATBALLS

CRUDITÉ PLATTER

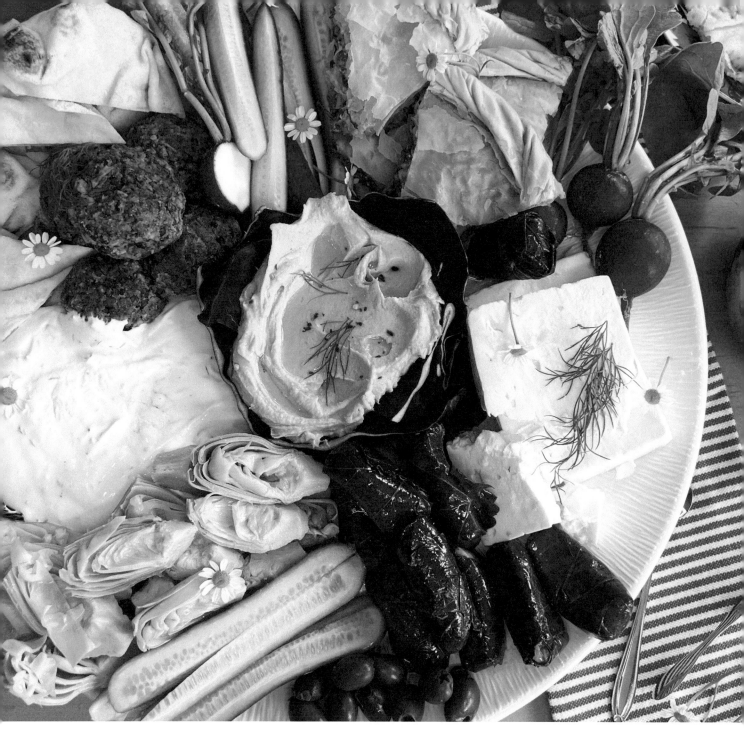

MEZZE PLATTER

SERVES 8

Everyone I know either likes or loves Greek food. What's not to love? It's always so healthy and the taste can't be beaten. Use a plant-based meatless ball like my delicious Chick Pea Lentil Balls (page 86) featured in the Dinnertime chapter of this book. Make them smaller to serve more like a bite-sized appetizer or larger to be stuffed inside a pita.

Make what you can in advance and buy the rest. Entertaining should be fun and not time-consuming. Use the cucumbers you grow in your garden for this eye-catching platter that will wow your guests. You can also make this for dinner and serve it as a grazing board, and everyone can pick and choose as they please.

NOURISH

INGREDIENTS:

- 15-20 Chick Pea Lentil Balls (page 86)
- 1 box frozen Spinach and Feta Spanakopita, store-bought
- Garlic Hummus (recipe follows)
- Tzatziki Dip (recipe follows)
- 1 (8-ounce) jar Kalamata olives
- 1 (10-ounce) package pita bread, cut into pieces
- 1 (8-ounce) package feta, cut into cubes
- 1 (12-ounce) bag radishes
- 2 (9-ounce) container stuffed grape leaves, store-bought
- 1 (14-ounce) package Persian cucumbers (or regular)
- 1 (12-ounce) jar artichoke hearts, drained
- 1 small head of red cabbage, use outer leaves
- Garnish: Mint leaves and lemon slices
- Large platter or wood board

Garlic Hummus:

- 1 (29-ounce) can chick peas, rinsed and drained (reserve a little liquid)
- 2 fresh garlic cloves
- 2 tablespoons tahini
- A good drizzle of extra virgin olive oil
- Ground sea salt
- Red chili flakes
- ½ lemon, squeezed (about 1 ½ tablespoons)
- Garnish: red chili flakes, crispy chick peas, olive oil, and dried parsley flakes
- High-speed blender (or food processor)

Tzatziki Dip:

- ½ cup shredded cucumbers
- 1 cup 2 % Greek yogurt
- 1 lemon, squeezed
- 1–2 tablespoons fresh dill, finely chopped
- Garlic powder to taste
- Sea salt to taste
- Cheesecloth

Make the Garlic Hummus.

Add the chick peas to the blender along with a little aquafaba liquid (about 3 tablespoons), garlic, tahini, a good drizzle of olive oil, sea salt, a dash of red chili flakes, and half of a lemon squeezed (about 1 ½ tablespoons). Blend at high-speed. Add more oil as needed, or even a splash of cold water, until you have achieved the desired creamy and smooth consistency.

Place the hummus inside a few large cabbage leaves, which will serve as a bowl. Add the garnish to jazz it up and make it visually appealing.

Note: Aquafaba liquid is the liquid the chick peas are soaked in. Reserving some of this and adding it to the hummus will make it extra creamy. You may also sauté the garlic to take away the strong flavor, add the garlic cloves to a pan with a drizzle of olive oil and sauté until translucent.

Make the Tzatziki.

Start by shredding the cucumbers, then strain them through a cheesecloth. Next, in a small bowl, add the Greek yogurt, lemon juice, shredded cucumbers, finely chopped dill, garlic powder, and salt to taste. Mix until well combined. Garnish with more dill and chill until ready to use.

Assemble the Platter.

Bake the Spanakopita according to the directions on the box. In the meantime, cut up the pita into triangles for easy dipping. Cut the mini cucumbers lengthwise or thinly cut regular cucumbers widthwise. Cut a few radishes in half, keep some whole. Cut the artichoke hearts into smaller bite-sized pieces.

Place the olives in a bowl. Add the bowl to the platter along with the hummus. Fan the pita around the hummus. You may add the chunks of feta to a bowl or use as fill in once the platter is assembled, same for the stuffed grape leaves. Add the remaining ingredients to the platter.

Right before serving, place the warmed Chick Pea Lentil Balls onto the platter by the Tzatziki Dip. The Spanakopita can go all around the edges of the platter. Garnish with mint leaves and lemon slices.

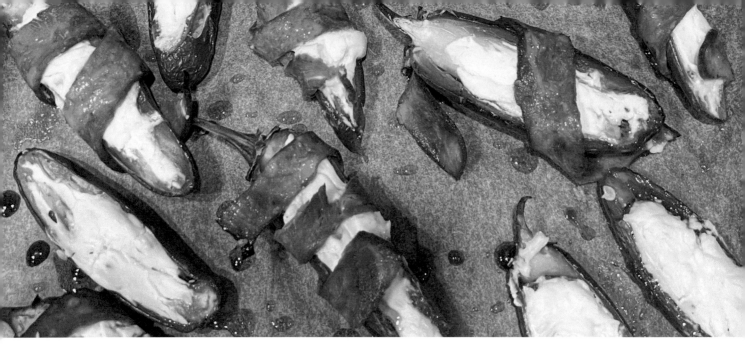

JALAPEÑO POPPERS
(Gluten Free)

=== MAKE 24 POPPERS ===

These jalapeno poppers are filled with a blend of 3 cheeses–Monterey Jack, cream cheese, and soft garlic and herb cheese. The Monterey Jack and cream cheese give these a slightly tangy flavor profile. The jalapenos are first roasted whole, then the seeds are scooped out. Next, the jalapenos are stuffed, then wrapped with bacon for visual appeal and a salty crunch. For a vegetarian variation, you may omit the bacon altogether and add some chopped fresh chives to the tops, and they are equally good.

These will disappear quickly, so make a double batch if these are for a party. Planting jalapeno peppers in your garden is a great idea, so you can make my Jalapeno Poppers on repeat all summer long. These will not disappoint.

INGREDIENTS:

- 12 large jalapenos, whole
- 1 cup light cream cheese, room temperature
- ½ cup Monterey Jack cheese, shredded
- 3 tablespoons soft garlic and herb cheese, room temperature
- Sea salt to taste
- 2 packages turkey bacon (or bacon), halved lengthwise
- Chili oil
- Garlic powder (optional)
- Narrow spoon

Preheat the oven to 400 degrees.

Rinse and dry the peppers. Place them onto a parchment-lined baking sheet. Bake for 15 minutes until softened and slightly charred. Once cool enough to handle, cut the peppers lengthwise and scoop out the seeds. Leave the stem intact for visual appeal. Set these aside.

In a small bowl, mix the cream cheese, Monterey Jack cheese, and softened garlic and herb cheese. Add sea salt to taste. Garlic powder is optional. Once it's to your liking, fill the peppers with the mixture using a narrow spoon.

Next, cut the bacon in half lengthwise. Wrap a piece around the peppers and place onto a baking sheet lined with parchment paper. If you are making these for a party, leave some without bacon for those living a vegetarian lifestyle.

The last step is to add a tiny drizzle of chili oil to each pepper. Bake in the oven for about 20 minutes until bacon is cooked through.

Everyone will love these! Great appetizer for a graduation party which is when I first made these. In the fall, these are also party-perfect for game day.

QUINOA AND BLACK BEAN BAKE
(Gluten Free)

INGREDIENTS:

- 1 cup dry tricolor or plain gluten-free quinoa (pronounced keen-wah), rinsed and drained
- 2 cups water
- 2 (15.5-ounce) cans black beans, rinsed and drained
- 1 orange or red bell pepper, diced
- 1 small red onion, diced
- 6–8 scallions, white and light green parts only
- Garlic salt to taste
- Chili pepper seasoning to taste
- Cayenne seasoning (optional)
- 5–6 tablespoons light cream cheese
- 1 lime, squeezed
- Non-stick cooking spray
- Medium-sized, oven-safe baking dish
- 3-quart pot with lid
- Large strainer
- Tortilla chips, for serving
- Garnish: sour cream, 1 diced tomato, hot sauce, and guacamole, or my Broccomole Dip (recipe follows)

Topping:

- 1 cup low-fat shredded cheddar cheese, part-skim mozzarella cheese (or Mexican cheese)
- 3–4 scallions, white and light green parts only, diced

Broccomole Dip:

- 3 large broccoli heads (2 ½–3 cups chopped broccoli stems, boiled, peeled, and chopped)
- 2 medium avocados
- A tiny drizzle of a good quality extra virgin olive oil
- 1 small chunk sweet yellow onion
- 1 fresh garlic clove
- 1 ½ limes, squeezed
- Ground sea salt to taste
- 2 slices medium red onion, diced
- High-speed blender

Preheat the oven to 375 degrees.

Rinse the quinoa before cooking it. Pour it directly into a large strainer and rinse well.

Then add the quinoa along with the water to the pot. Add the black beans, peppers, red onion, scallions, and seasonings. Stir until well combined.

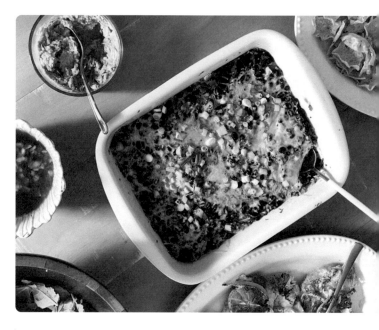

Note: Taste the black beans before adding them to the pot. If they need salt, add it; otherwise, this will impact the taste of this dish. Also, I have substituted cannellini beans in this recipe, which work well. If you use these, add them after you cook the quinoa, as they will break if cooked too long.

Next, heat the mixture on medium-high. Allow it to come to a boil then add the lid and reduce it to a simmer for about 15 minutes, or longer until quinoa is softened. Follow box directions. It is done when all the liquid is completely absorbed, and the quinoa is translucent with a noticeable rim around it. It will also be very fragrant from the peppers which really make this dish amazing.

Pour the mixture into the greased baking dish, swirl in the cream cheese, and add the lime juice. Allow it to cool slightly and taste it. Be sure the seasonings are to your liking. Then flatten out the top and add the shredded cheese and more diced scallions to the top.

Bake at 375 degrees for 10 minutes until the cheese melts. Then top with tomatoes and serve with sour cream, guacamole, or Broccomole. If you like it spicy, add hot sauce.

This is a great appetizer, or you may serve it for dinner alongside some pan-fried tortillas.

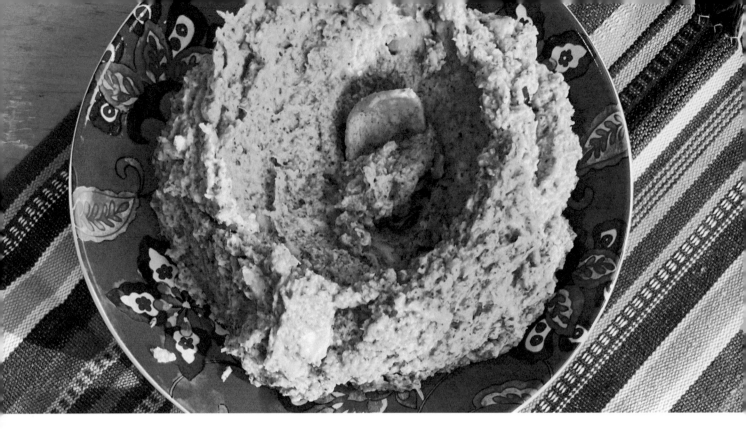

BROCCOMOLE
(Gluten Free)

We love everything about guacamole except the price of avocados and the fact that the dip always browns after an hour or so. This is my popular Broccomole which is a spin-off of guacamole. I swap out half of the avocados for broccoli. It tastes delicious and stays green for a few days in the fridge. This is a game-changer.

I have tested this recipe far too many times, and as a result I can tell you it's amazing. It tastes like authentic guacamole, and it's lump-free, as I avoid the broccoli florets and focus on the tender and delicious broccoli stems, which are often discarded. As a former volunteer chef in a homeless shelter who taught residents how to avoid food waste and use what's in the pantry and fridge, I like to be creative and use what I can.

A few tips. . . be sure to add lots of lime and ground sea salt—that is the key to this fabulous dip. We use salted tortilla scoops to devour this dip, which is eaten in minutes, so make 2 batches. If you want to opt for a heathier alternative to chips, use steamed or roasted broccoli florets to scoop up the dip. Alternatively, use the broccoli florets to make my Broccoli Pizza (page 111)

Make the Broccomole.

Boil the broccoli heads in a large pot until they are just fork tender, but still bright green. Once done, rinse under cold water to retain that gorgeous color, part of the charm of this dip. Next, let this cool. Then cut off the florets and hold for another night or use for dipping into this fabulous dip alongside salty tortilla chips!

Next, peel off the outer layer of stems as best as possible, it doesn't have to be perfect. Then chop into chunks and measure 2½–3 cups of stems. Add them to the high-speed blender or a food processor.

Then scoop out the insides of 2 ripened avocados and add to the blender along with a tiny drizzle of olive oil. Toss in a small chunk of sweet yellow onion and garlic, this will impart some extra flavor into the dip because broccoli doesn't have much flavor. Pulse for 2 minutes using the agitator stick. Once creamy and lump-free, add the mixture to a bowl.

Next, add in the lime juice and ground sea salt. Then finely dice 2 slices of red onion and hand mix the dip. Taste it and adjust seasonings to your liking.

MINI GOAT CHEESE AND PROSCIUTTO PIZZAS

MAKES 16 MINI PIZZAS

My Italian friends tell me these pizzettes or mini pizzas are popular in Italy. These can also be made with pastry dough, another great option.

INGREDIENTS:

- 1 package biscuits, 8 large biscuits (or gluten-free biscuits)
- 1 (4-ounce) package of goat cheese, warmed
- 8 slices halved, Prosciutto di Parma
- Hot honey or regular honey
- Salt to taste
- Garnish: Thyme sprigs

Preheat the oven to 375 degrees.

Cut the biscuits in half horizontally, making 16 biscuits. Place them onto a parchment-lined baking sheet.

Take the goat cheese out of the package. Place on a microwave-safe plate and warm for 5 seconds in the microwave. The cheese is much easier to spread onto the biscuits warm. Next, Spoon 2 teaspoons of goat cheese onto the biscuit and spread evenly. Bake the biscuits partially for 10 minutes.

Cut the prosciutto in halves widthwise and add to the top of the pizza rounds once they have baked for 10 minutes. Bake an additional 6 minutes or longer until golden. Follow package directions to be sure the biscuits are cooked through, test one.

Take them out and add a tiny drizzle of hot honey (or regular honey). Broil for 1 minute to crisp up the prosciutto. Alternatively, you may add the prosciutto after they have fully baked for 16 minutes. I prefer the prosciutto crispy. Garnish with some thyme leaves. Salt to taste.

These are a great snack or appetizer and would look beautiful on a food board.

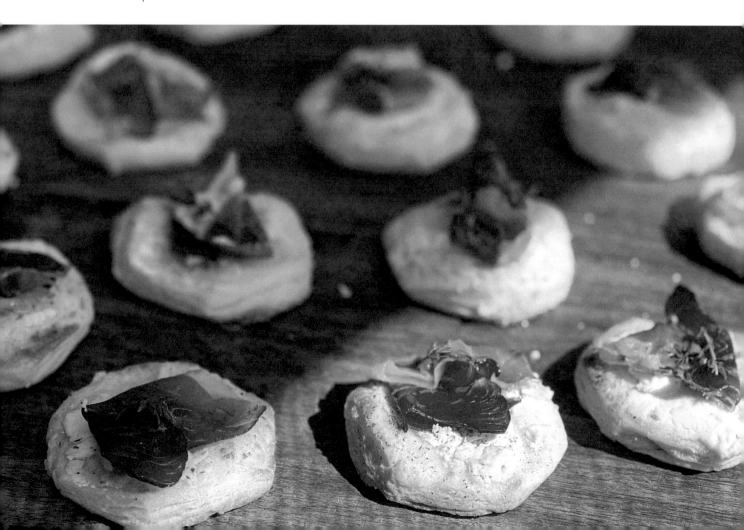

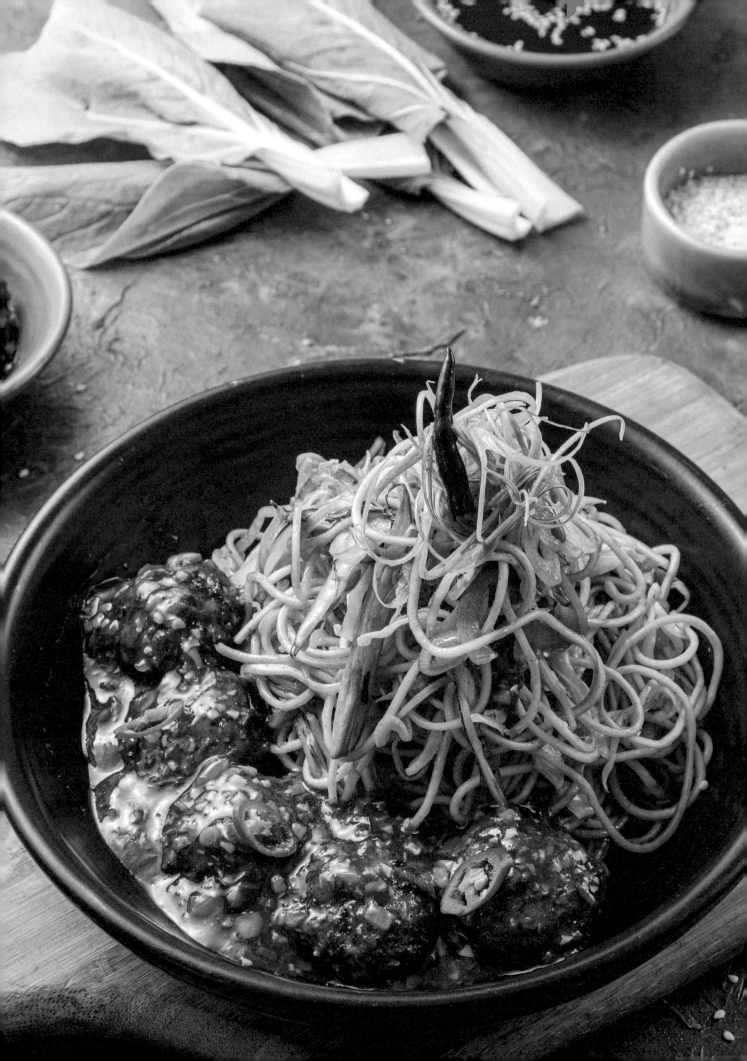

MINI TURKEY MEATBALLS

YIELDS 40 MINI MEATBALLS

These are a huge hit at parties. They are a similar combination as the Asian-Inspired Meatballs in the Dinnertime section of this book, but with a few adjustments. This recipe does not have any breadcrumbs, making it easily adaptable for a gluten-free lifestyle. I make these in advance of a party or family gathering and freeze them. Then I defrost them in the fridge overnight. I prepare the sauce fresh, add in the defrosted meatballs, and heat on low. So delicious!

INGREDIENTS:

- 2 lbs. lean ground turkey meat (85% or 90% lean)
- 4 tablespoons low-sodium soy sauce (or gluten-free soy sauce)
- 2 tablespoons hoisin sauce (or gluten-free hoisin sauce)
- ½ tablespoon garlic powder
- Sprinkle of red chili flakes and ginger powder (or freshly grated ginger, about 2 teaspoons)
- Salt and pepper to taste
- Drizzle of chili oil (optional)
- Large non-stick frying pan

Sauce:

- ¼ cup hoisin sauce (or gluten-free hoisin sauce)
- ½ cup soy sauce (or gluten-free soy sauce)
- ⅛ cup honey
- Freshly grated ginger, about 1 teaspoon
- Red chili flakes
- Water to loosen

Toppings:

- Scallions, diced
- Sesame seeds

Preheat the oven to 350 degrees.

In a large bowl, combine the turkey, soy sauce, hoisin sauce, garlic powder, red chili flakes, ginger, and salt and pepper to taste. Combine with clean hands.

Make 40 mini meatballs. Place them onto 2 parchment-lined baking sheets.

Bake about 20–22 minutes until cooked through.

Make the Sauce.

In a large non-stick frying pan, add the hoisin sauce, soy sauce, honey, freshly grated ginger, and red chili flakes. Add water to loosen (about ¼ cup). Heat on low for 10 minutes.

Once the meatballs are done, add them to the pan with the sauce. Cover the meatballs in the sauce, keeping heat on low. Top with sesame seeds and chopped scallions. Simmer for 15 minutes until flavors meld together.

Reference foodsafety.gov for safe internal cooking temperatures for meat, fish, pork and poultry. Always use an instant-read thermometer to be sure food is cooked to safe internal temperatures.

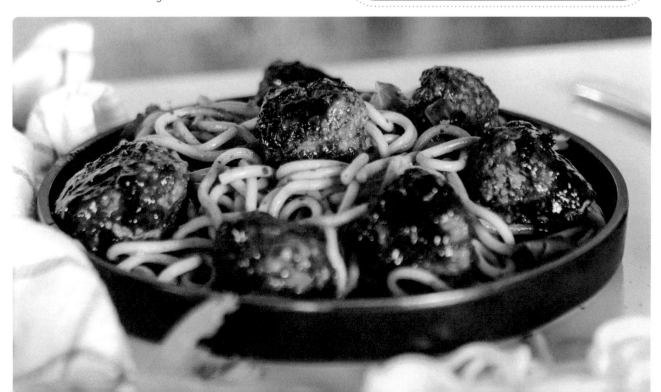

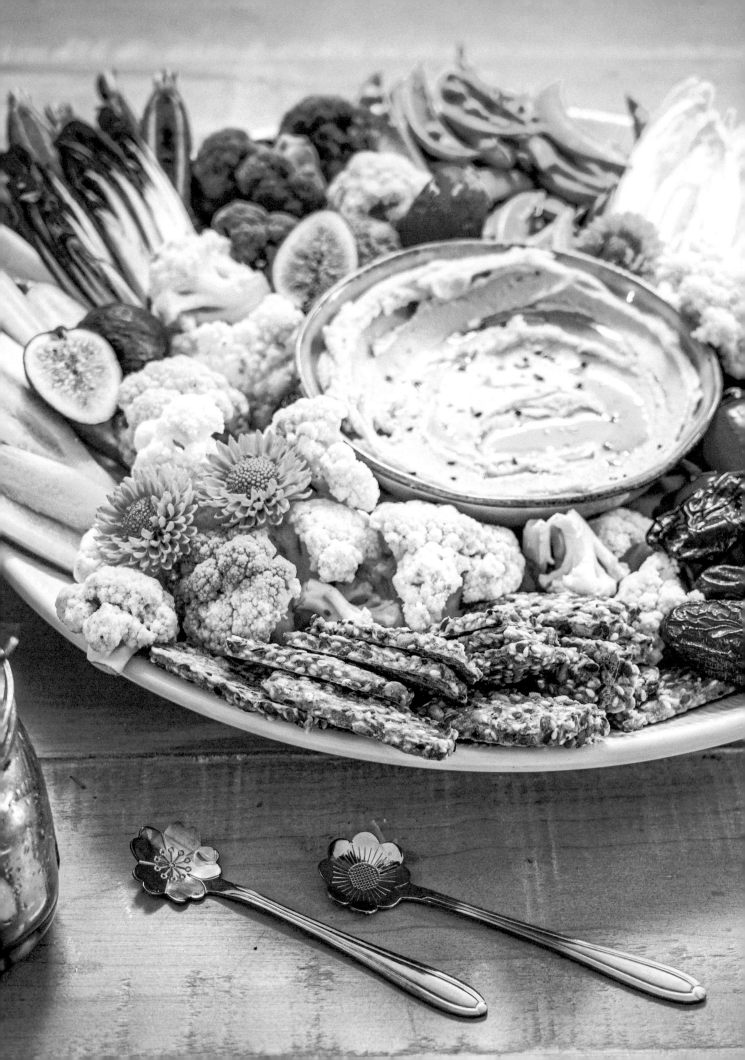

CRUDITÉ PLATTER

SERVES 6

INGREDIENTS:

- Hummus (store-bought or homemade Garlic Hummus (page 37)
- 1–2 heads cauliflower, florets only (orange, purple, or white)
- 1 bag sugar snap peas
- 3 heads endives (yellow and purple), quartered lengthwise
- 1 bunch purple and yellow carrots, peeled and halved lengthwise
- 8–10 small red peppers, whole
- 10 medjool dates, pitted
- Seeded crackers (recipe follows) (or gluten-free crackers)
- Black mission figs, halved (optional)
- Garnish: radishes and food-safe flowers
- Medium-sized round platter or wood board

Seeded Cracker Ingredients:

- ¼ cup whole wheat flour plus 1 tablespoon, and more for dusting (or super-fine almond flour)
- 1 tablespoon unsalted and roasted sunflower seeds
- 1 tablespoon Zen Basil Seeds (or chia seeds)
- 2 tablespoons ground flaxseeds (or flax meal)
- 1 tablespoon sesame seeds
- 1 tablespoon everything bagel seasonings
- Sprinkle garlic powder
- ½ cup boiling water
- Extra sunflower seeds and sesame for topping cracker
- Sprinkle of sea salt (optional)
- Rolling pin

Making the Seeded Crackers.

In a medium-sized bowl, add the dry ingredients including seasonings (reserve 1 tablespoon of flour). Add the boiling water to the bowl, mix, and let the cracker dough rest 10 minutes. It's as simple as that!

Note: A gluten-free alternative would be to use a super-fine almond flour instead of whole wheat flour. Be sure to first whisk the almond flour to break up any clumps. The crackers have a buttery, melt in your mouth texture and taste great.

In the meantime, preheat the oven to 350 degrees.

After 10 minutes and once cooled, add 1 more tablespoon of flour to the dough and mix it with clean hands. Then place it onto a piece of parchment paper on a wood board to spread the mixture. Top it with a tiny sprinkle of flour and the second layer of parchment paper.

Next, using a rolling pin, roll the cracker dough out as thin as possible, about ¼-inch thick. This is an important step. Gently peel off the parchment paper and top with more sunflower and sesame seeds, about 1 tablespoon of each. Be sure to press them into the cracker dough. Topping with sea salt is an option.

Holding the ends of the parchment paper, gently place the cracker dough onto a narrow baking sheet. Bake for 40–45 minutes until browned.

Baker's tip: The crackers are done when they feel hard. If you notice any soft spots, break the soft spots off and re-bake for an additional few minutes, or until they are crisp. If you didn't roll out the cracker dough evenly, this will happen. You want them to crunch when you bit into them. Practice makes perfect.

Harvest tip: Purple cauliflower gets its beautiful purple jewel-toned hue from the presence of the antioxidant anthocyanin, which is also found in red cabbage and red wine. Orange cauliflower comes from a genetic mutation that allows the plant to hold more beta carotene. Orange and purple cauliflower are higher in antioxidants than white cauliflower. Peak harvest season in the northeast is in the Fall months. You'll find these at local farmer's markets.

Assembling the Rainbow Platter.

Start by adding the bowl of hummus to the center of the platter and building the other ingredients around it. Split some of the peas in half to expose the inside. Set a small bowl out with salt for dipping radishes. Place one inside the bowl so people get the idea of dipping. If figs are in season and you can find them, use them. Be sure to cut them in half to expose the gorgeous inside. This adds visual interest and appeal to your platter. Food-safe flowers add a nice decorative touch.

Nutrition tip: Eating a diet that is abundant in fruit, colorful vegetables, and legumes like chick peas or sugar snap peas is good for our brain health, according to Samara. Learn more about other foods that aid in brain health in the Q & A section with Samara at the end of this book.

Food waste tip: Refrigerate any leftover veggies and roast them the next day to avoid food waste.

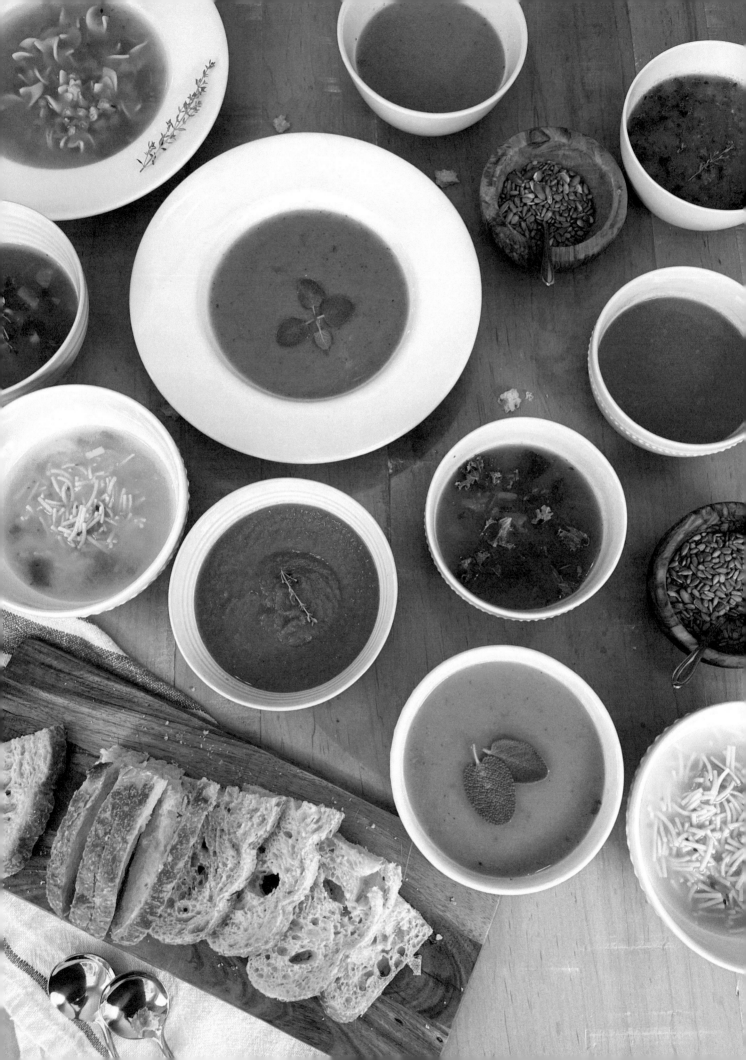

SOUPS AND SALADS

ORANGE AND FENNEL SALAD
(Gluten Free)

SHREDDED CHICKEN AND LEEK SOUP

EGGLESS CAESAR SALAD
WITH ARTICHOKES AND HEARTS OF PALM

CREAMY CAULIFLOWER SOUP
(Gluten Free)

BUTTERNUT SQUASH SOUP
(Gluten Free)

BURRATA SALAD

ORANGE AND FENNEL SALAD
(Gluten Free)

This is a next-level salad with chopped baby kale, orange slices, thinly sliced fennel, chopped fresh dill or fennel fronds, and pomegranate seeds paired with a creamy citrus-garlic dressing. It's a wonderful combination for spring or summer when we are keeping things simple and light.

INGREDIENTS:

- 3–4 Cara Cara Navel Oranges, peeled and cut into slices, then halved
- 1 bulb fennel, thinly sliced
- 1 (16-ounce) bag baby kale, chopped
- 1 bunch fresh dill (or fennel fronds)
- 1 pomegranate, seeds only

Citrus-Garlic Dressing:

- 2 pink oranges (Cara Cara Navel Oranges), squeezed, juices only
- ½ small lemon, squeezed
- ½ cup extra virgin olive oil
- ½ cup sherry vinegar (or apple cider vinegar)
- ½ teaspoon honey mustard
- 1 small fresh garlic clove
- 1 tablespoon chopped yellow onion
- Salt and pepper
- Water as needed, can use a little as a substitute for less oil
- High-speed blender

Make the Dressing.

Prepare the dressing in a high-speed blender. Add all the above ingredients and purée until a creamy texture is achieved. This process is called emulsion. You combine two or more unmixable liquids (like oil and vinegar/lemon juice) through agitation (like whisking or blending) to create a uniform and homogeneous mixture, in this case a dressing. A little food science! Chill the dressing in the fridge until you are ready to toss and serve the salad.

Prepare the Salad.

Thinly slice the oranges and fennel. A good chef's knife is helpful. Chop the baby kale. Chop a small handful of dill, or you can use the fennel fronds. You can add as much or as little as you like for this salad, or store some in the fridge for another use.

Fun fact: Fennel fronds, the tops of the fennel bulb, can be used like an herb to impart fennel's licorice notes in raw and cooked dishes. Fennel is related to the celery family.

I prefer the underwater method for releasing the pomegranate seeds. Cut the pomegranate into quarters and submerge the pieces in a bowl filled with water. Break pieces to release the seeds, which will drop to the bottom and the pulp (white inside part) will float. Discard the white parts.

Be sure to wash all fruit and vegetables before consuming to rid it of any possible bacteria and pesticides. Any time you're cutting into fruit or vegetables with a skin or rind, you take the chance of introducing bacteria and chemicals from the surface and contaminating the inside. Soaking fruits and vegetables in apple cider vinegar and thoroughly rinsing them is a good way to properly clean your fruits and vegetables. Use 2 tablespoons vinegar per 8 cups of water added to a bowl. Soak fruits and thick-skinned vegetables like peppers and avocados for 10 minutes.

Assemble the Salad.

The salad will have chopped baby kale as its base, orange slices, fennel slices, a sprinkling of chopped dill, and a few tablespoons of pomegranate seeds. Serve the dressing on the side or toss right before serving. Sliced almonds are a nice addition. Garnish with a wedge of pomegranate for a decorative touch.

Harvest tip: Pomegranate harvest season usually runs from mid-September through to late December or even early January in some regions of North America. Pomegranates contain an antioxidant that is also noted for many other health benefits.

Kale is a superfood that is high in vitamins and minerals. Did you know that kale is related to the cabbage family

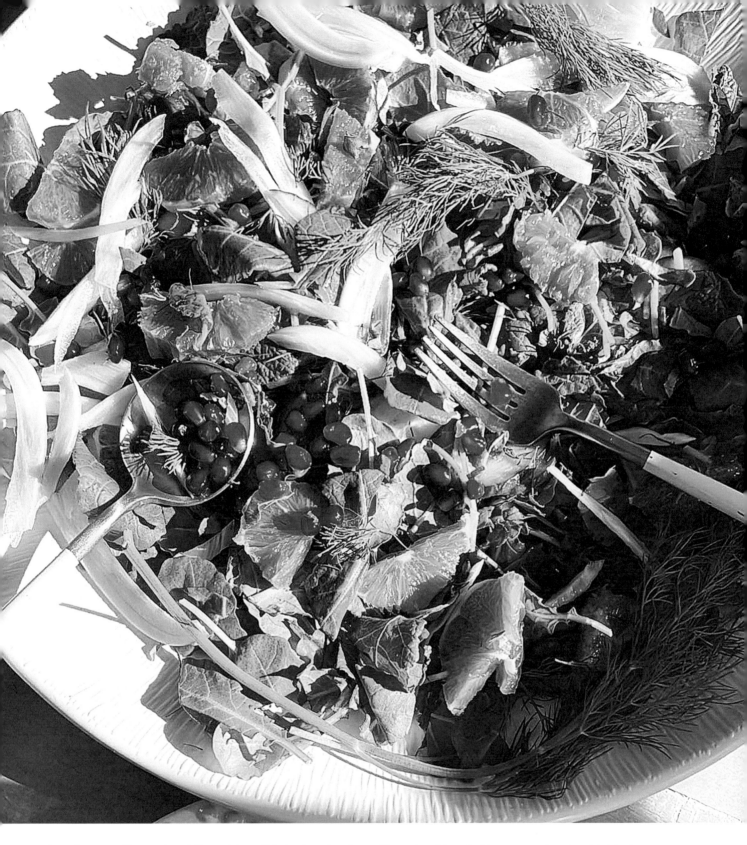

but does not form a head like cabbage? It is also closely related to collard greens. Kale is known for its thick, sometimes tough leaves, so it can be helpful to tenderize the large leaves with some lemon juice prior to serving in a salad. The baby kale can simply be tossed in a vinegary dressing and will be ready to eat.

To make this salad into a meal, pair with black-pepper-encrusted citrus salmon. Start by marinating the salmon in orange and lemon juices and a drizzle of honey. Then add a generous amount of cracked black pepper to the salmon, when baked it will create a coating. Roast until it's crispy and cooked through. Always use an instant-read thermometer to check for safe internal temperature.

SHREDDED CHICKEN AND LEEK SOUP

INGREDIENTS:

- 2 large leeks, cut widthwise, light green and white parts only
- 2 shallots, cut into slices (or 1 medium yellow onion)
- 1 cup combined fresh parsley and fresh dill, loosely packed
- 2 tablespoons salted butter
- 2 cups Yukon potatoes, cubed (about 1 medium potato)
- 2 containers chicken stock
- 3 tablespoons all-purpose flour (or 1-2 tablespoons cornstarch)
- 2 cups roasted and shredded chicken breast (or rotisserie chicken, white meat only)
- 1 cup low-fat milk
- ¼ cup heavy cream (optional)
- Salt and cracked black pepper
- A good quality extra virgin olive oil
- Large pot with lid

Thinly cut the leeks widthwise and soak in water for 5–10 minutes. Drain and soak again until water runs clear. Thinly slice the shallots or yellow onion.

Soak the herbs in water until the water runs clear. You can use a large handful for this soup. Feel free to adjust to your tastes. You can use only parsley, or I have used cilantro. Let your palate be your guide. Next, finely chop the herbs. Set them aside.

Add the butter to the pan and heat the leeks for 10 minutes on medium-low until softened. Add a pinch of sea salt. Next, add the onions and heat for an additional 5–8 minutes.

In the meantime, peel the potato and dice it into cubes. Add the cubed potatoes to the pot with a drizzle of olive oil and a pinch more of salt.

Add the 1 ½ containers of stock to the pot, reserve a little. Whisk in flour (or cornstarch) to thicken soup. If you prefer it more liquidy, skip the flour.

Shred the cooked chicken and add about 2 cups into the pot. Add the chopped herbs. For a vegetarian option, double the potatoes and use vegetable stock–equally as good! On low heat, add the slightly warmed milk and cream, for a creamier soup. Season the soup with cracked black pepper and salt to taste. Simmer for 1 hour or longer. Garnish with some crispy bacon and a swirl of cream.

Fun fact: Leeks are members of the onion family. They grow long thick stems or "shanks" instead of bulbs like onions. They retain a fair amount of dirt, so always cut them and soak them in a bowl of water.

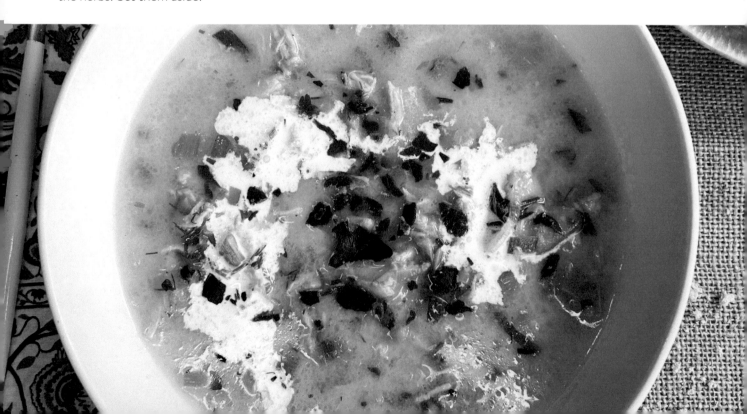

ALL THINGS BLOOM IN TIME

It's that time of year
I peek outside my kitchen window
And see the abundance in my garden
It seems to have happened overnight
I run to pick the ripened eggplant and fragrant basil
My tomatoes are always late to bloom
Sometimes staying green until late August
Cucumbers and zucchini tend to steal the sunshine
Overpowering and shading the most
Magnificent fruit in the garden
I cut them back dramatically and say every summer
That I won't plant cucumbers and zucchini again
But summer comes and I do
Soon the tomatoes will be in full bloom
I will make sauce and celebrate them
For now, I'll make eggplant parmesan and zucchini fritters
cucumber salad and pesto
All things bloom in time

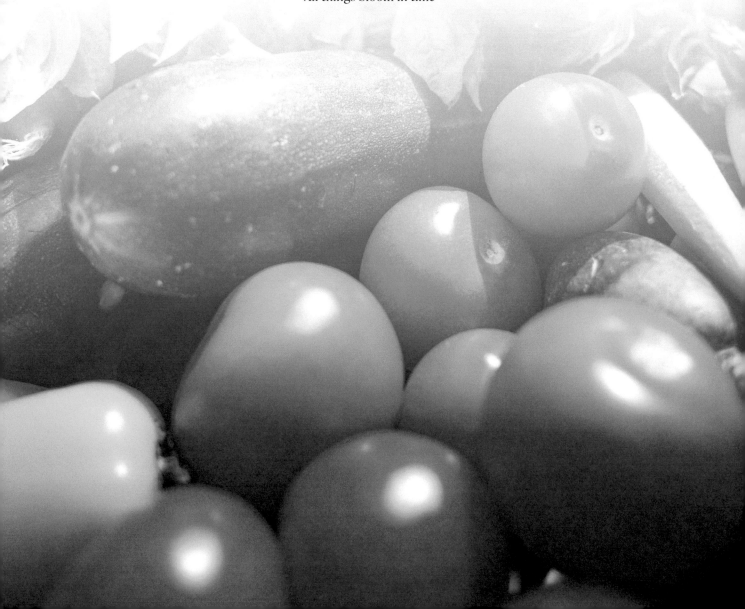

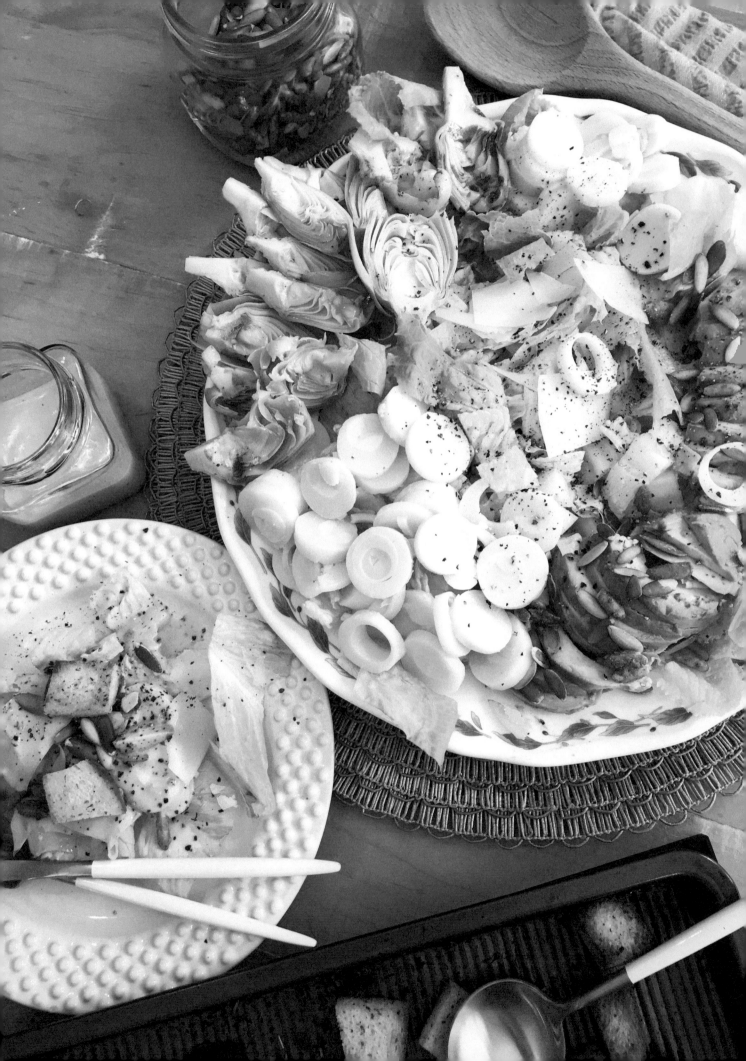

EGGLESS CAESAR SALAD
WITH ARTICHOKES AND HEARTS OF PALM

This is a very visually appealing salad that tastes amazing with the addition of homemade herby croutons and zesty eggless Caesar dressing. Add some chicken or salmon to make this heartier and dinner is served. This is a show-stopping salad, so make this for your next family or friend gathering. I prefer serving this on a platter for a gorgeous presentation, but tossing all the ingredients together in a big bowl works great too.

INGREDIENTS:

- Herby Homemade Croutons (recipe follows):
- 3 romaine hearts, chopped
- 1 (12-ounce) jar grilled and marinated artichoke hearts, drained (quartered)
- 1 (14-ounce) can hearts of palm, thinly sliced widthwise
- 2 avocados, sliced
- ¼ cup salted and roasted pumpkin seeds
- ½ cup shaved Parmigiano-Reggiano (or parmesan cheese)
- Crack black pepper to taste
- Large round platter (or wooden bowl)

Herby Homemade Croutons:

- 4 slices of thick white bread, cut into chunks (or gluten-free bread)
- A good quality extra virgin olive oil
- 2 teaspoons Herbes De Provence seasoning
- Garlic powder (optional)

Eggless Caesar Dressing:

- ½ cup extra virgin olive oil
- 1–2 lemons, squeezed
- 2 teaspoons minced garlic
- 1 teaspoon anchovy paste in a tube (or more)
- 1 teaspoon spicy brown mustard
- 2 tablespoons capers plus 2 tablespoons brine
- ½ cup finely grated Parmigiano-Reggiano (or parmesan cheese)
- Cracked black pepper to taste
- Sea Salt to taste
- Whisk
- Mason jar with lid

Preheat the oven to 375 degrees.

Make the Croutons.

Cut the slices of bread into cubes. Keep the crust on the bread – that's the best part! In a bowl, toss the bread with a drizzle of olive oil and the herbs. Then dump the bread onto a baking sheet lined with parchment paper.

Bake for 15 minutes, then put the oven temperature up to 400 degrees to crisp and brown them for a few more minutes, roughly 4 minutes. Keep an eye on them so they don't burn.

In the meantime, while you are baking the croutons, wash and dry the lettuce. Then chop it into bite-sized pieces. Place the lettuce onto the platter. If you are using heads of romaine, discard a few of the outer layers.

For this recipe, I used grilled and marinated artichoke hearts, but if you can't find them grilled, that is fine. Use what is available, marinated, or in water works. Thoroughly drain and cut them into quarters.

Place the artichokes on top of the romaine along the outer edge of the platter. This creates a nice design element.

Next, drain the hearts of palm and cut into slices widthwise. Place on the bed of lettuce and disperse throughout.

Next, slice the avocado. A good tip is to cut it on a wood board, in half lengthwise, discard the pit, and slice inside the shell, before scooping out the flesh with a large spoon – keeping it intact and together as best as possible. Place the avocados on the bed of lettuce.

Last, right before serving salad, add the pumpkin seeds for a bit of a crunch.

Make the Eggless Caesar Dressing.

In a bowl, combine the olive oil, juice of 2 lemons, minced garlic, anchovy paste, mustard, capers, sea salt, and cracked black pepper. Whisk until well combined. Mash the garlic and capers with the back of a spoon. Then add the freshly grated cheese. Alternatively, if you can find garlic paste in a tube, that works great in this dressing. Pour the dressing into the mason jar and chill until ready to serve.

Shake dressing right before serving and drizzle over the salad. Sprinkle on more cracked black pepper and top with shaved parmesan cheese. Add croutons after dressing is poured. Leftover croutons will last in an airtight container on the counter. Refrigerate leftover salad and dressing.

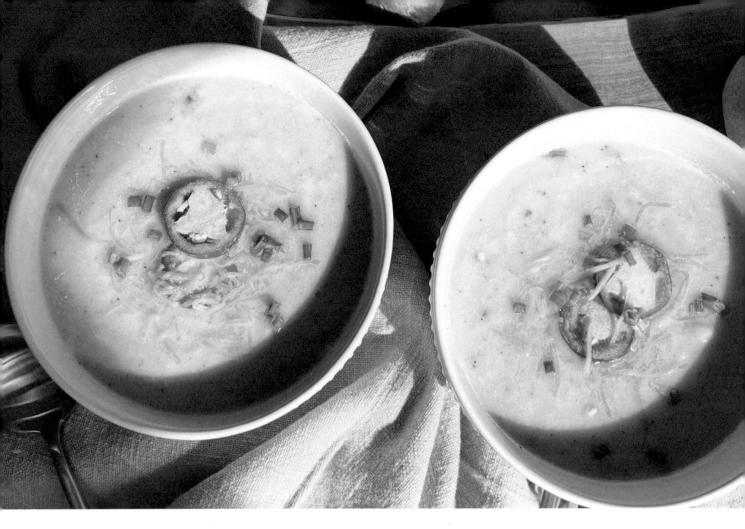

CREAMY CAULIFLOWER SOUP
(Gluten Free)

SERVES 4-6

INGREDIENTS:

- 2 tablespoons salted butter
- 2–3 tablespoons extra virgin olive oil
- 2 shallots, diced
- 1 ½ heads cauliflower, steamed (about 11 cups of florets)
- 4 cups water plus more as it thickens
- 1 ½ teaspoons onion powder
- Garlic salt to taste
- Salt and cracked black pepper to taste
- ¼ teaspoon or more red chili flakes
- 1 large jalapeño, diced with seeds and a few slices for garnish
- 1 cup milk low-fat (or regular milk), warmed
- 1 ¼ cups finely shredded mild cheddar cheese
- 3 tablespoons chopped fresh chives
- High-speed blender
- Large pot

Sauté the onions in butter and olive oil on medium-low heat for 8 minutes. Then add the onions to the blender along with cooled steamed and drained cauliflower florets and 2 cups of water. Do this in 2 batches, adding more water as needed. Blend twice for the creaminess texture.

Add the mixture to the pot with remaining water. Season with onion powder, garlic salt, cracked black pepper, and salt to taste.

Stream in milk slowly and whisk continuously so it doesn't curdle. Keep the heat on simmer. Add the finely shredded cheese and stir until it starts to melt. Last, add the chopped jalapeño with (or without) seeds and chives.

Allow soup to simmer for about 45 minutes (or longer), adding water as needed to loosen.

Garnish with more cheese, jalapeño slices, and fresh chives. Serve with warm out of the oven Olive Loaf Bread (page 121).

BUTTERNUT SQUASH SOUP
(Gluten Free)

Butternut squash soup is on repeat all fall and winter long. I will change it slightly each time. Sometimes instead of sweet potato, I will add pumpkin. I make a big batch of this soup and store it in large glass mason jars in the fridge for easy eating throughout our busy week. Serving with crusty Italian bread (or gluten-free bread) makes this a hearty meal that the whole family will love.

INGREDIENTS:

- 2 lbs. butternut squash, cut and diced
- A good quality extra virgin olive oil
- 6 fresh sage leaves, whole
- 1 large shallot, diced
- 1 cup sweet potato or yam (about 1 medium potato)
- 1 (48-ounce) container chicken stock (or vegetable stock)
- 2–3 thyme sprigs
- Sea salt and black pepper to taste
- A pinch of freshly grated nutmeg and a splash of cream (optional)
- Large pot
- High-speed blender

Chef tip: Use only good quality extra virgin olive oil. It will make or break your soup. Same holds true about your stock. To test the olive oil, dip some bread in it. If there is no aftertaste, you may use it in your soup.

Preheat the oven to 400 degrees.

Place cubed squash onto a parchment-lined baking sheet. Roast in the oven for about 40 minutes until fork tender.

In the large pot, drizzle a small amount olive oil and add a sprinkle of sea salt. Add the sage leaves. The sage will infuse an amazing flavor base into your soup. Next, sauté the diced shallots until translucent. Discard the sage leaves or save a few as garnish.

Add the squash into the pot with the onions and mix them together. Allow them to cool a few minutes before adding to the blender.

In the meantime, cook a sweet potato (or yam) in the microwave until a fork can pierce through it easily. Alternatively, you may roast the sweet potato when you roast the butternut squash if you are not pressed for time. Let it cool. Scoop out the potato and measure about 1 cup, adding it into a small bowl.

Into the high-speed blender (mine holds 6 cups), add the cooled squash, and shallots along with 1 cup or more of chicken stock. Blend until the ingredients are puréed, and no lumps are present. Then add in the cooked sweet potato. Blend until smooth, adding more stock as needed to loosen.

Transfer the purée back into the large pot and add more chicken stock. I will typically use ¾ of a 48-ounce container for this recipe. As the soup thickens, you will add more, so keep it on hand. Refrigerate leftover stock for the next day.

Next, add a few sprigs of thyme or any fresh herbs (you may discard after 1 hour or so). Add salt and pepper to taste and a drizzle of olive oil. A pinch of nutmeg is always a good idea.

Simmer on low heat for about 1 hour and serve with warmed Italian bread. Try my Olive Loaf Bread featured in this book.

As a garnish, you may sauté more sage leaves and add them on the top of your soup for a visually appealing bowl of heartwarming soup or top with pumpkin seeds. Feel free to swirl in a little cream into each bowl.

Seal any leftovers in an airtight container in the refrigerator for up to 3 days.

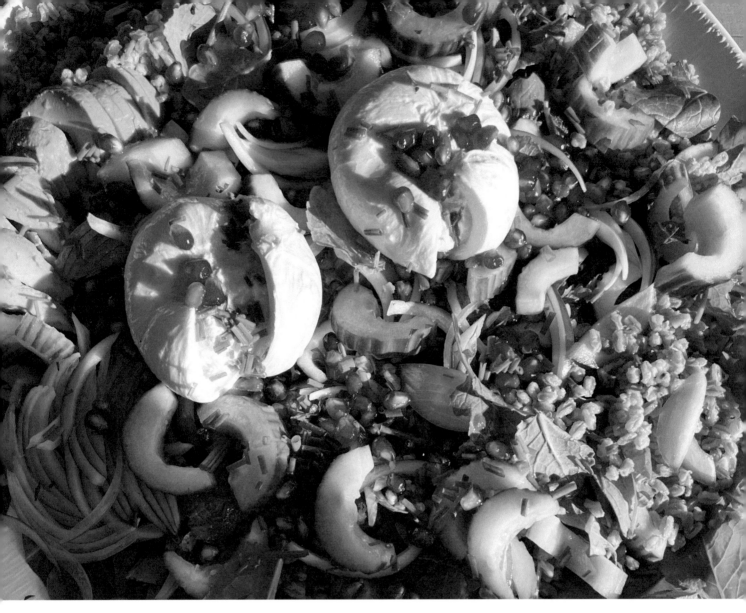

BURRATA SALAD

SERVES 4

INGREDIENTS:

- 8 cups chopped curly kale, chiffonade (or chopped baby kale)
- 1–2 lemons, squeezed
- ¼ cup fresh parsley, chopped
- 2–3 cups cooked farro, warm
- 1 large English cucumber, seeded
- 1–2 large avocados, pitted and sliced
- 1 large pomegranate, seeded
- ½ cup Pickled Red Onions (recipe follows)
- 3 tablespoons fresh chopped chives
- 1 (8-ounce) package burrata (2 large bulbs)
- Drizzle extra virgin olive oil
- Large platter

Red Wine Vinegar-Pomegranate Dressing:

- ½ cup red wine vinegar
- ¼ cup extra virgin olive oil
- 1 tablespoon pomegranate molasses (or honey)
- Salt to taste
- Pomegranate seeds (optional)
- Mason jar with tight-fitting lid

Pickled Red Onions:

- 1 large red onion, thinly sliced
- 1 cup water
- 1 cup vinegar (distilled white vinegar and apple cider vinegar combined)
- 3–4 tablespoons granulated sugar
- 4 garlic cloves
- Peppercorns and garlic salt
- Small pot
- 2 (8-ounce) jars with tight-fitting lids

Make the Pickled Red Onions.

These are best after 1 day (or longer), but I have made them the same day I make this salad and used them after about 3–4 hours of soaking, and they are still very good. A good chef's knife will ensure that the slices are thinly cut.

In the small pot, add 1 cup of vinegar and 1 cup of water. I use a combination of apple cider vinegar and distilled white vinegar. You can even use some rice vinegar. Add 4 tablespoons of sugar and bring the water to a slight boil. Allow the sugar to evaporate, then add the onions and cook for a few minutes until softened. Allow the onions to cool and add to the mason jars. Refrigerate once cooled.

Use pickled red onions to elevate meals like sandwiches, pulled pork burritos, salads, and more. Bring these to friends and family gatherings as a hostess gift.

Prepare the Salad.

Pull all the leaves off the kale stem. Place them inside a large bowl with cold water and soak for 5 minutes. Dry on a clean dish towel. Then finely chop the leaves or cut into chiffonade–also known as ribbons.

In a large bowl, add the kale and the juice of 1–2 lemons. This will serve to soften the kale leaves, which can be very tough. Do not skip this step. Mix well with clean hands. Let this sit on the counter for about 1 hour or longer.

Next, soak the parsley in cold water. Rinse and soak about 3 times. Dry on a clean dish towel. Sometimes parsley and other herbs can hold a fair amount of dirt. Cut off the stems for this salad. If you are using them to cook, it's a good idea to keep them intact as they have a lot of flavor. Finely chop the parsley and measure about ½ cup, loosely packed. Set it aside.

After the kale has soaked up the lemon juice about 1 hour, make the farro according to package directions. You want to top the kale with the warmed farro because it will slightly wilt the greens. Add chicken or beef bouillon to add flavor to the water or cook the farro in stock. Reserve 3 cups of farro for this recipe.

While the farro is cooking, cut the cucumber in half lengthwise and scoop out the seeds with a narrow spoon and discard. Cut ½-inch pieces using a knife or crinkle cut them. On a wood board, cut the avocados in half, slice inside the shell, and scoop out with a spoon. Last, extract the seeds from 1 pomegranate. I prefer the underwater method for extracting the seeds, which is described under the Orange and Fennel Salad.

Prepare the Red Wine Vinegar-Pomegranate Dressing.

In a small bowl, combine the red wine vinegar, olive oil, and pomegranate molasses. Salt to taste.

Assemble the Salad.

Add the kale ribbons to a large platter. Then top with chopped parsley, cucumber slices, and pickled onions. Add the warm farro right before serving, and top with chopped chives. Add the avocado slices, burrata bulbs, and toss in the pomegranate seeds. Cut into the burrata bulbs and add a tiny drizzle of olive oil.

Dress the salad with the Red Wine Vinegar-Pomegranate Dressing, or any vinaigrette, or balsamic glaze. I love this salad just as much with my homemade Balsamic Glaze.

Make the Balsamic Glaze.

In a small pot, add 2 cups of good quality balsamic vinegar, bring to a boil and simmer for 15 minutes until reduced to half. I promise you do not need any sugar in this recipe and the taste is so sweet!

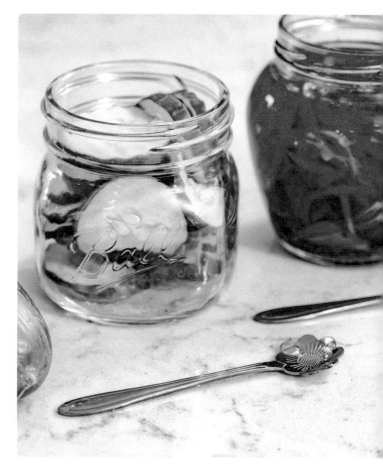

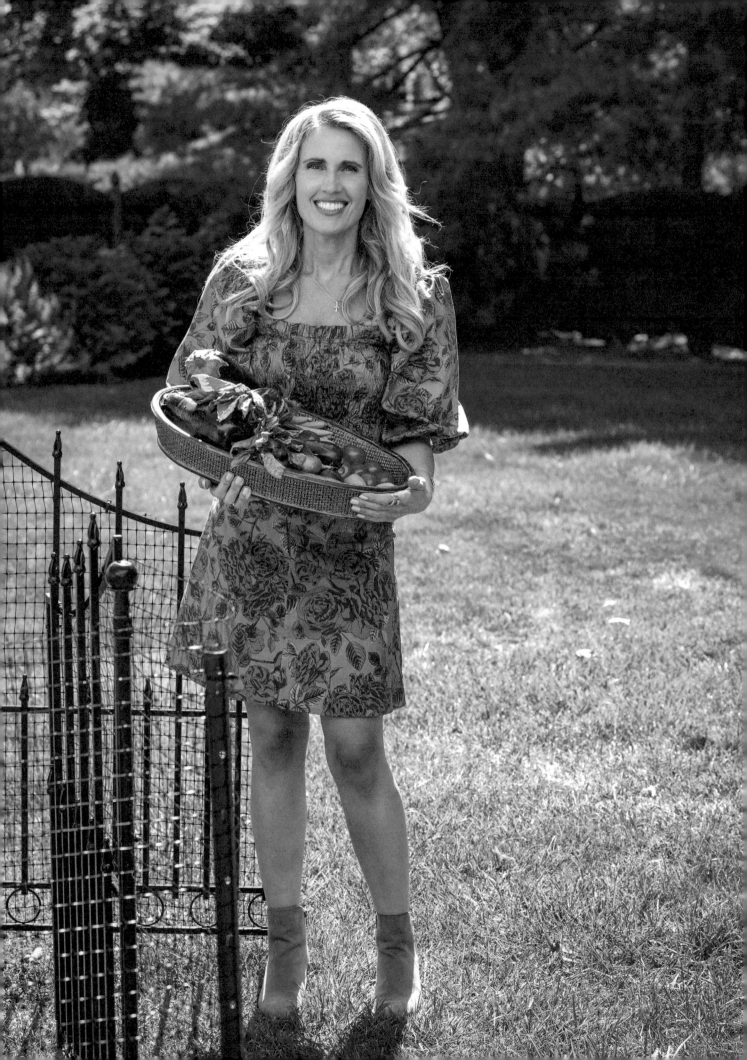

VEGETABLE MAINS AND SIDES

SPICY ASIAN-INSPIRED CRISPY CAULIFLOWER BITES
WITH HONEY-CHILI GARLIC SAUCE
(Gluten Free)

EGGPLANT THREE WAYS
(Gluten Free)

SPICY POTATOES
(Gluten Free)

FRITTERS AND VEGETABLE PANCAKES

MEXICAN STREET CORN ON THE COB
(Gluten Free)

COLLARD GREEN VEGGIE WRAPS
WITH SEARED TOFU
(Gluten Free)

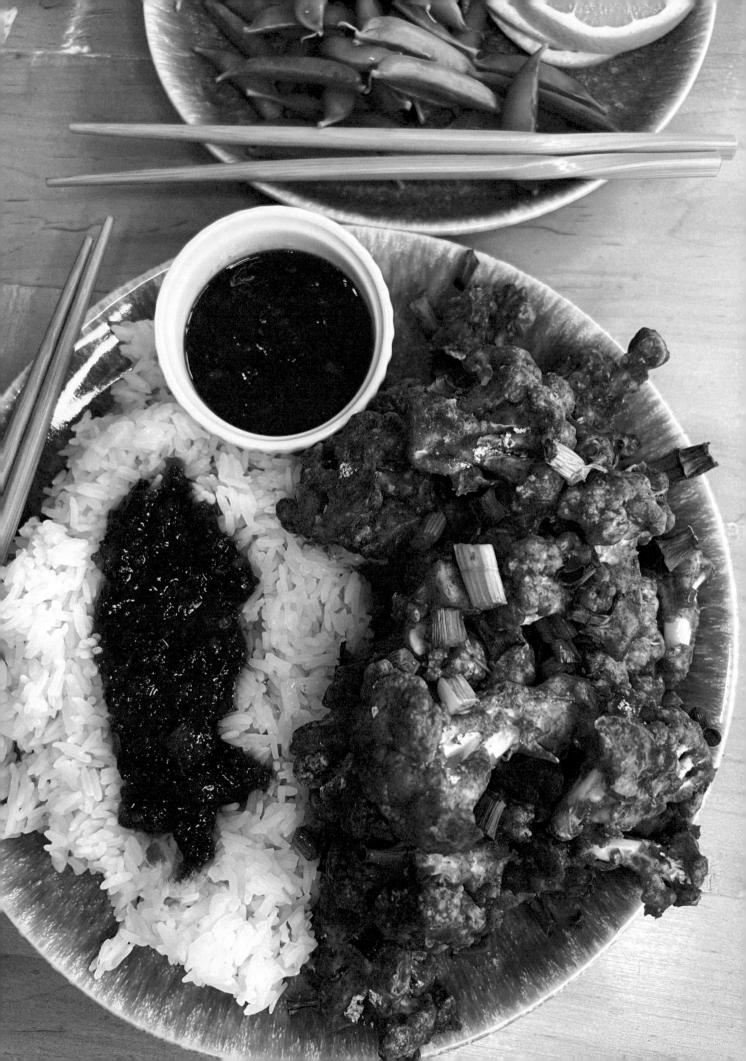

SPICY ASIAN-INSPIRED CRISPY CAULIFLOWER BITES
WITH HONEY-CHILI GARLIC SAUCE
(Gluten Free)

This is a family favorite and a wonderful main meal that everyone will enjoy. Pair with fluffy jasmine rice, orange slices, and warmed sugar snap peas (my favorite!).

INGREDIENTS:

- 1 medium-sized Chinese cauliflower head, cored
- 1 cup cornstarch
- 2 large eggs
- 3 teaspoons paprika (plus 1 teaspoon added to oil to coat)
- ⅓ cup extra virgin olive oil
- 4 tablespoons hot sauce or more
- 1 bunch scallions, diced (reserve some for sauce)
- Sea salt
- 2–2.5 Q metal bowls for mixing
- 3 cups Jasmine rice, cooked

Honey-Chili Garlic Sauce:

- ¼ cup honey
- 2 tablespoons extra virgin olive oil (or preferred oil)
- 2 teaspoons freshly grated ginger
- 1 teaspoon rice vinegar
- ⅓ cup gluten-free chili garlic sauce (found at Asian or Korean markets)
- 3 tablespoons chopped scallions
- 1–2 teaspoons hot sauce (optional)
- Water as needed to loosen
- Small non-stick frying pan

Preheat the oven to 400 degrees.

While holding the cauliflower head with two hands, stem down, knock the cauliflower head on a wood board twice to dislodge the core. Whatever remains intact, cut off the florets. It's a quick and simple way that gets the job done. Cut longer stems of cauliflower florets down. Be sure pieces are somewhat bite-sized for easy eating.

Add ½ cup of cornstarch (reserve the rest) in 1 bowl, and 2 premixed eggs in other bowl. Add the florets into the bowl with the cornstarch and toss to fully coat. Then toss the cornstarch-coated florets into the premixed egg mixture and mix with a spoon (or clean hands) to fully coat.

To the bowl that had the cornstarch, add the remaining ½ cup of cornstarch, along with 3 teaspoons paprika (reserve the rest), and a good sprinkle of sea salt. Mix with a fork to combine. Next, add the egg-coated florets back into the paprika-cornstarch mixture and toss to combine. They should be fully coated.

Rinse 1 bowl and add the olive oil, hot sauce, and 1 teaspoon paprika. Last, toss the now paprika-cornstarch-coated florets with the olive oil/hot sauce to give it extra flavor. Be sure all the florets are completely covered.

Add the florets and diced scallions to a parchment-lined baking sheet and bake for 30 minutes, turn halfway through.

Make the Sauce.

In a small non-stick frying pan, add the honey and heat on low. Then add the olive oil, grated ginger, rice vinegar, chili garlic sauce, and water to loosen. Last, add the scallions. The hot sauce is optional. Add water as needed to loosen sauce.

You may fully coat the cauliflower bites with the sauce or set it in a bowl for dipping.

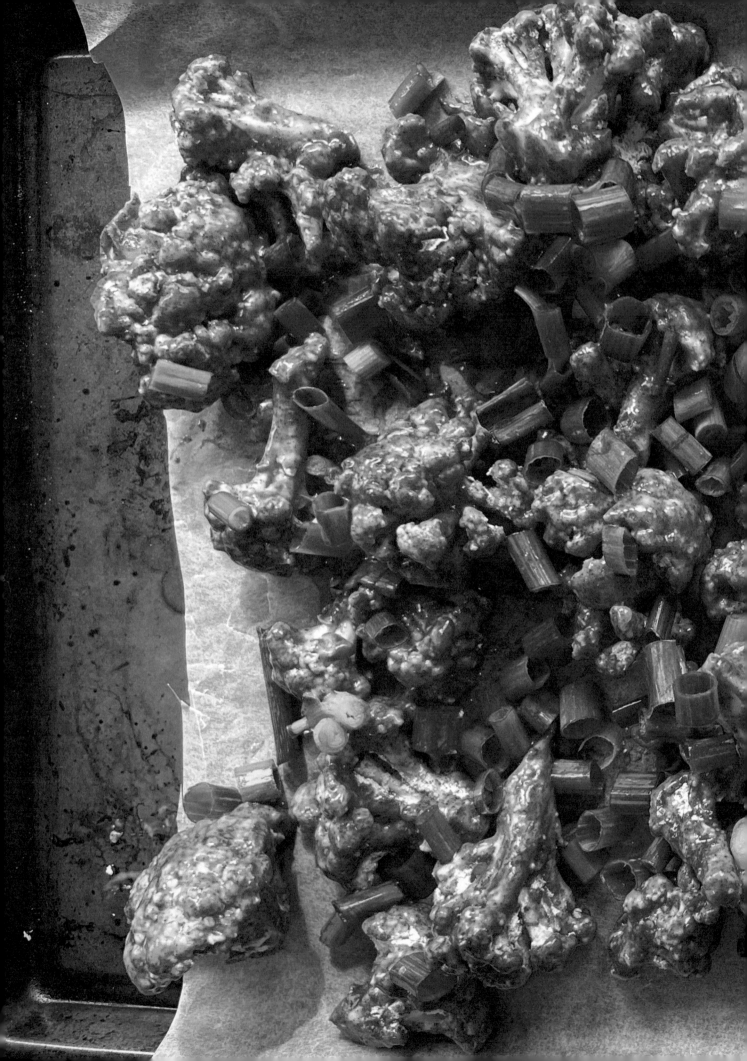

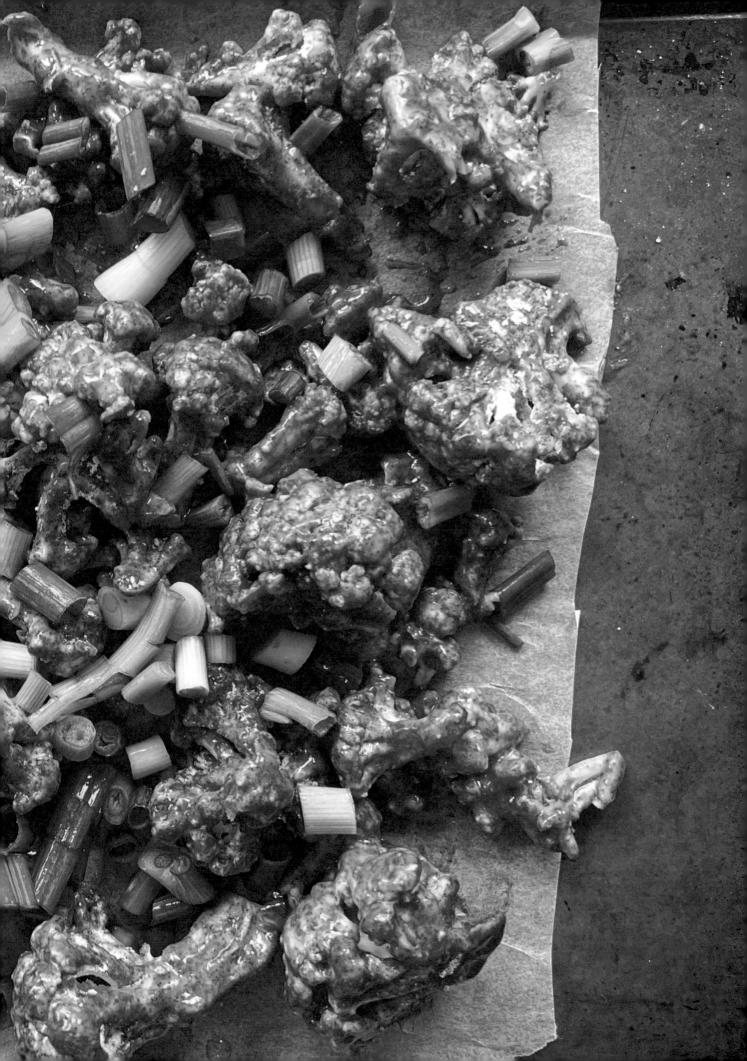

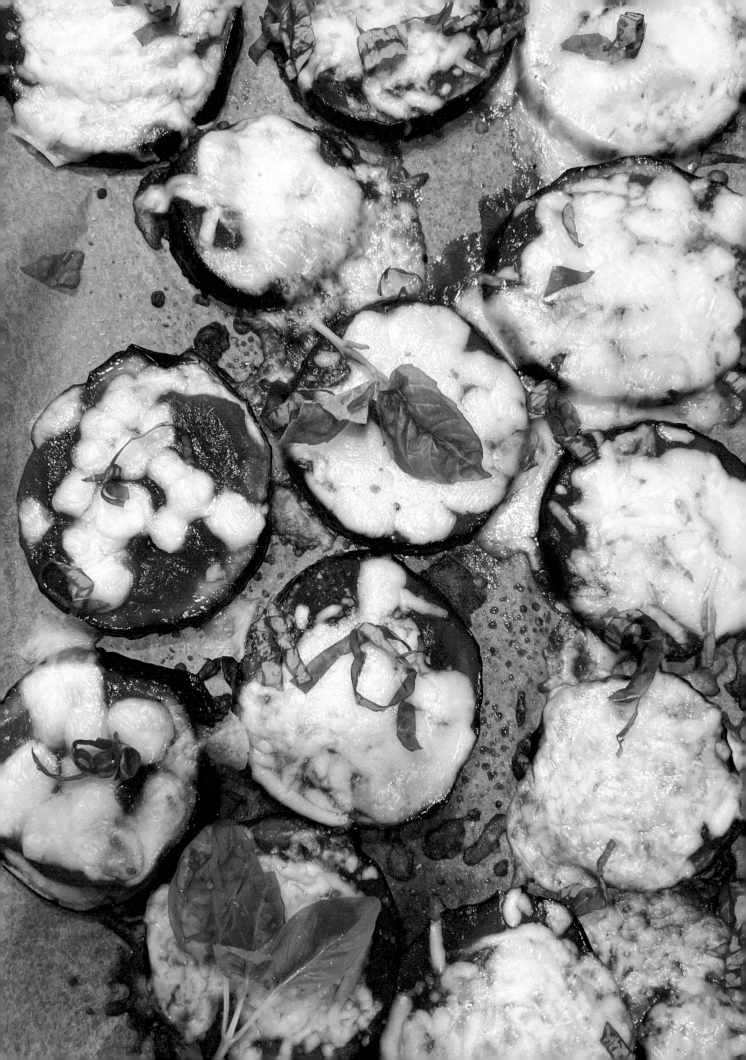

HEALTHY EGGPLANT PARMESAN
(Gluten Free)

INGREDIENTS:

- 1 large eggplant (or 2 medium), cut into 1-inch slices (about 8 slices)
- ½ jar prepared (or homemade tomato sauce)
- ½ cup shredded part-skim mozzarella cheese (or packaged mozzarella, finely diced)
- Dried Italian seasonings (or dried oregano)
- Garlic powder to taste
- Sea salt to taste
- Garnish: Fresh basil, cut into ribbons or torn, about 4–5 leaves
- Non-stick cooking spray
- Non-stick baking sheet

Grab those eggplants from your garden and make this super-easy, healthy, and delicious eggplant parmesan.

Preheat the oven to 425 degrees.

Rinse and pat the eggplant dry. Cut off the stem. Then cut 1-inch slices widthwise. If you prefer to peel the eggplant, feel free to do so, then cut it into slices. Depending upon the size of your eggplant, some are very large, you may have more than 8 slices. Always a good idea to get an extra eggplant because sometimes they are brown inside and you will not want to use that.

Sprinkle the eggplant slices with a little sea salt. After 15 minutes, pat it dry. Add the eggplant slices to a parchment-lined baking sheet. Spray each slice with cooking spray.

Roast the eggplant in the oven for 25–30 minutes, or until fork tender. Oven temperatures may vary. Flip the slices over hallway and spray again. If you made more than 1 tray, alternate trays on the racks so they cook evenly. Top each slice with 1–2 tablespoons of sauce, 2 tablespoons of cheese, a tiny sprinkle of seasonings, and garlic powder – a little goes a long way.

Place the eggplant back into the oven and lower the temperature to 400 degrees to melt the cheese, about 8–10 minutes.

Top each slice with sea salt and fresh basil torn or cut into thin ribbons.

Enjoy this as an appetizer or double the recipe to make it a heartier meal. Top with mini pepperoni slices and make eggplant-pepperoni pizza. Pile the eggplant onto some fresh Italian bread to make an eggplant parmesan sandwich. Great for summertime entertaining.

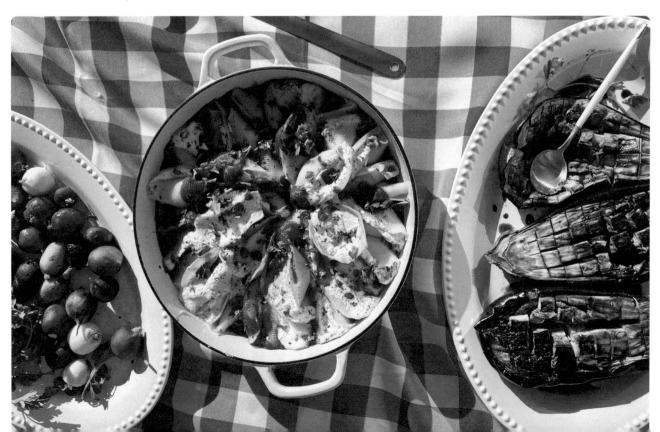

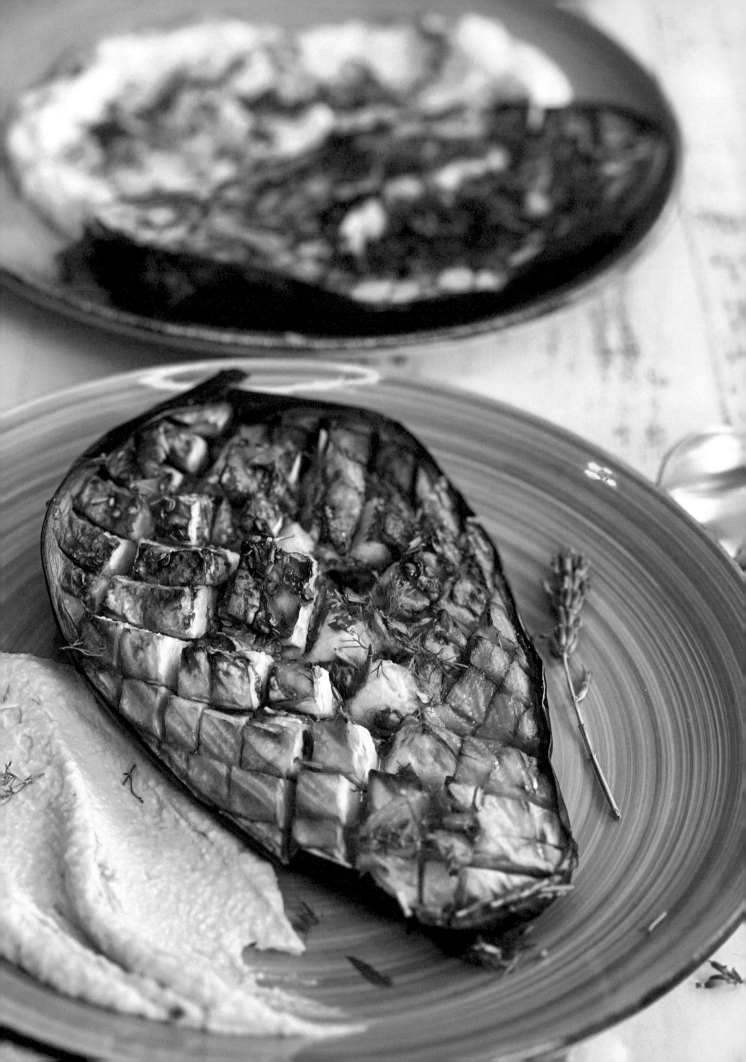

ROASTED EGGPLANT GRID

SERVES 4

INGREDIENTS:

- 2 medium eggplants
- A good quality extra virgin olive oil
- Sea salt to taste
- A drizzle of honey (or hot honey)
- Non-stick cooking spray

Preheat the oven to 450 degrees.

Prepare the Eggplant.

Rinse and pat the eggplant dry. Cut the eggplant in half lengthwise. With the eggplant skin side down on a cutting board, very carefully, cut a grid pattern in the flesh of the eggplant. Try not to cut all the way through the skin. Make shallow cuts. Salt and pat dry after 15 minutes.

Next, place the eggplant onto a baking sheet. Spray the eggplant thoroughly with non-stick cooking spray or drizzle with olive oil. Roast in the oven for 25 minutes (or longer) until golden brown.

Serve at room temperature with a drizzle of honey. Sydney loves it this way. Whipped ricotta would pair well with this, my Tzatziki Dip (page 37), or tahini on the side. Serve alongside a classic Italian dish like stuffed shells or spaghetti and meatballs.

Dining al fresco in the summer months is always a great idea. Feel free to change this recipe and try using the zucchinis from your garden, cut lengthwise. In this case, add some homemade pesto with fresh basil from your garden.

As I was quoted in the article "The Joy of Picnics" in the Summer 2022 issue of *Princeton Magazine,* "A picnic to me is a chance to become grounded in the literal and figurative sense. You become engulfed by the beauty of nature's landscape and awaken your sense of smell (fragrant flowers, ocean breezes), sense of sound (birds chirping, ocean waves crashing), and taste (yummy picnic food). It's an awe-inspiring backdrop that we cannot find anywhere else except in nature's midst."

ROASTED EGGPLANT SLICES

SERVES 4

INGREDIENTS:

- 1 large eggplant, thinly sliced
- Non-stick cooking spray
- Sea salt to taste

Preheat the oven to 425 degrees.

Thinly slice eggplant widthwise into ¼-inch slices. Add the eggplant slices to a parchment-lined baking sheet. Spray with non-stick cooking spray.

Roast for 20 minutes until browned and tender. Season with sea salt to taste.

We love these so much, especially in the summer months when cooking is lighter and more simplified. Dip in my homemade Garlic Hummus (page 37).

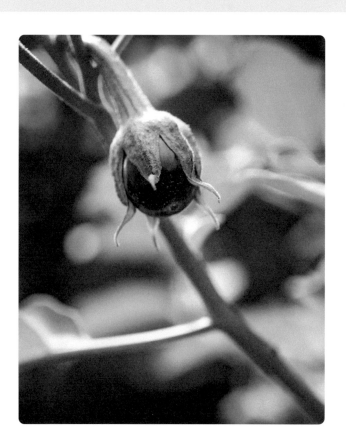

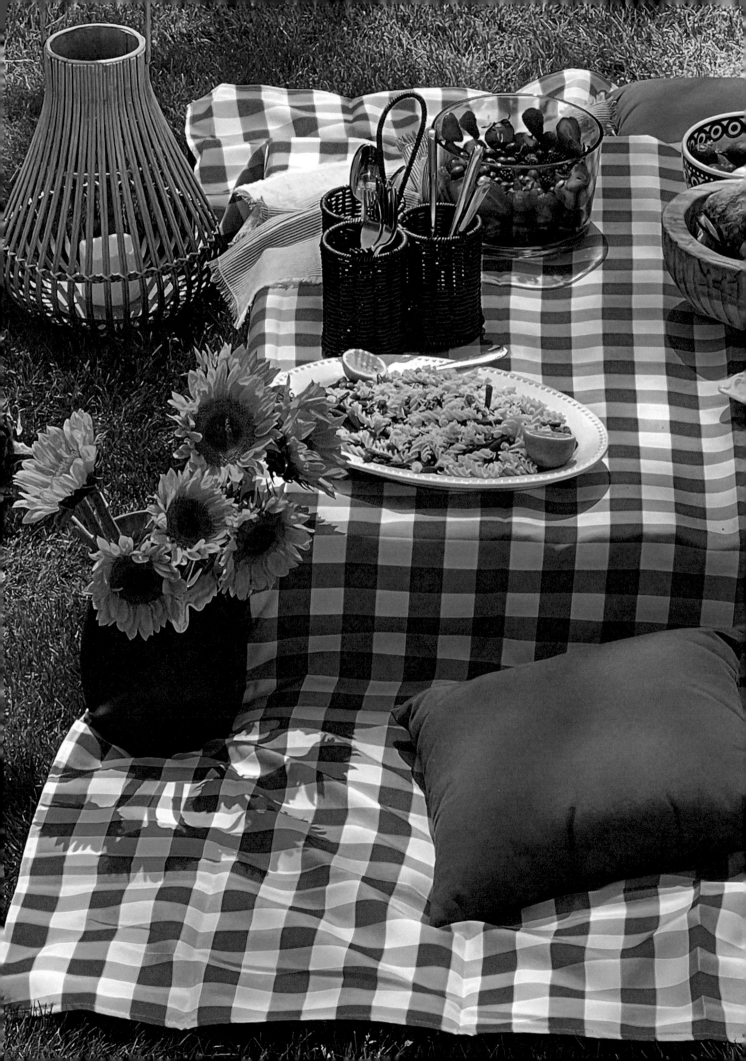

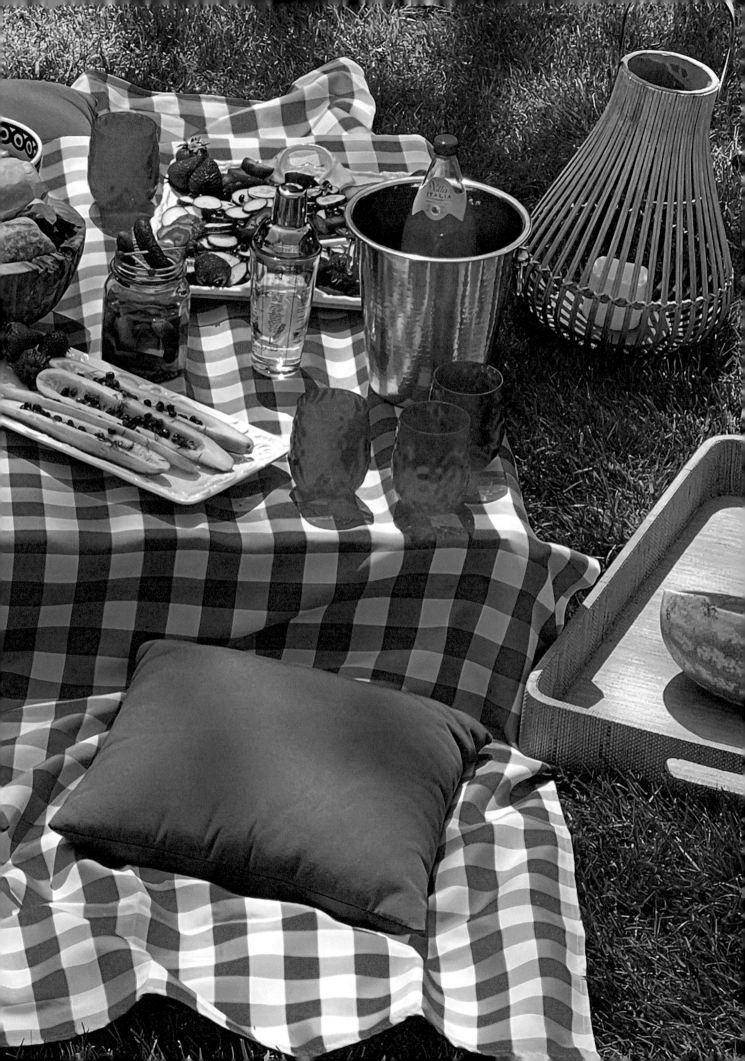

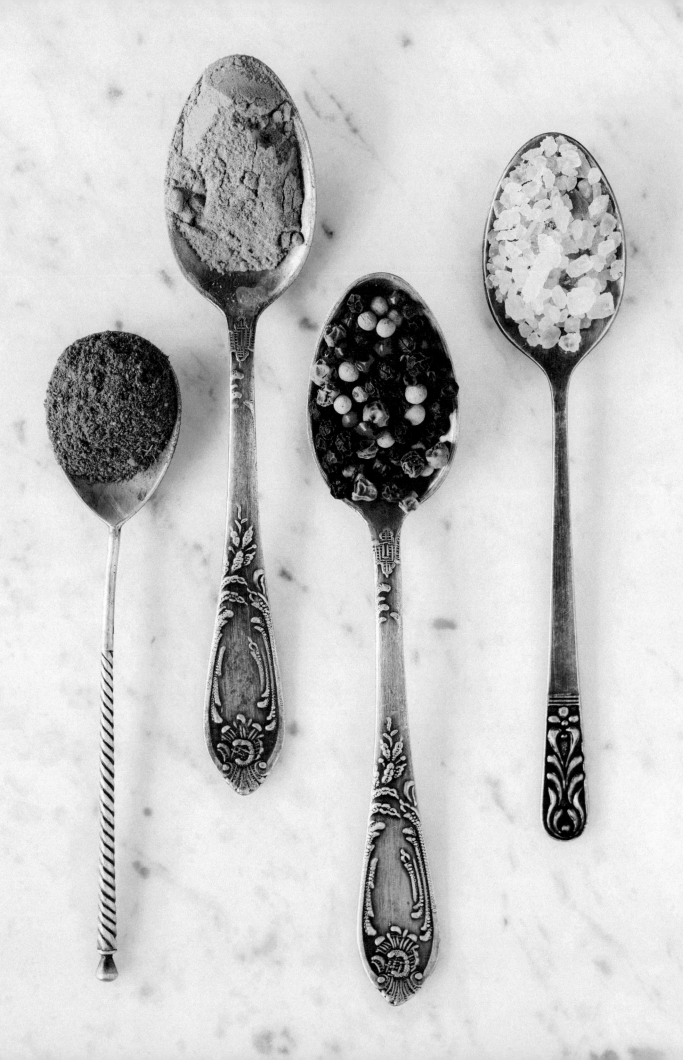

SPICY POTATOES
(Gluten Free)

INGREDIENTS:

- 3–4 large Russet (or Yukon potatoes), scrubbed and cut into bite-sized chunks (or mini potatoes halved or quartered)
- ½ cup extra virgin olive oil
- Coriander, paprika, black pepper, and parsley flakes to taste
- Ground sea salt to taste
- 2 tablespoons fresh parsley (or cilantro), chopped
- Cayenne pepper and red chili flakes (optional)
- Garnish: Freshly chopped parsley (or cilantro)

Preheat the oven to 425 degrees.

Wash and scrub the potatoes and cut into bite-sized chunks.

Add the potatoes to a large pot and bring them to a boil. Once fork tender, drain in a colander.

In a large bowl, add the following ingredients in generous amounts: olive oil, coriander, paprika, pepper, parsley flakes, and salt. If you like to kick up the heat and make it spicy, add a few tiny dashes of cayenne pepper. This really intensifies the spicy factor in these potatoes.

Whisk the ingredients to create a sauce. Add the potatoes and toss in the mixture. Add more paprika and black pepper once mixed.

Add the coated potatoes to a parchment-lined baking sheet. Add a dash of red pepper flakes (gives a little heat without overpowering it like cayenne) and more parsley flakes.

Place in the oven for 30 minutes, halfway toss potatoes. Then add more ground sea salt once done.

The potatoes should be crunchy on the outside, soft on the inside, and hold their shape. They have the texture of a french fry. Garnish with freshly chopped parsley or chopped cilantro.

Serve with a combination of sour cream, yogurt, and a squeeze of lemon. Add some spices and fresh chopped parsley. This will cool your palate from the spices.

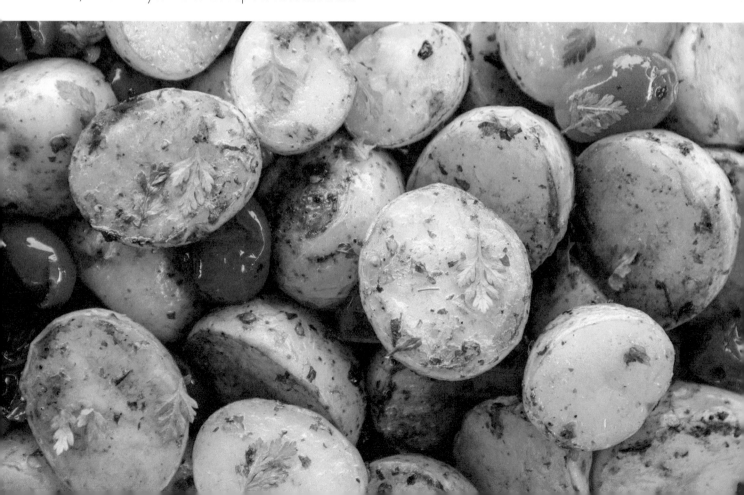

CARROT FRITTERS

Carrots are an excellent source of vitamin A, which is essential for eye health and good vision. They are high in fiber and good for digestion. I buy a large bag of organic carrots weekly and use them in various recipes. My kids love carrot fritters, carrot fries, carrot and ginger soup, and dipping carrots in my homemade hummus.

INGREDIENTS:

- 2 ½ large carrots, peeled and grated (yields about 2½–3 cups)
- 4 scallions, diced
- 4 tablespoons all-purpose flour (or rice flour)
- ½ cup panko Italian-style breadcrumbs (or gluten-free breadcrumbs)
- 2 large eggs
- ½ tablespoon dried parsley flakes
- ¼ teaspoon paprika
- Ground sea salt and black pepper to taste
- ¾ cup shredded mozzarella
- A good quality extra virgin olive oil
- Medium-sized non-stick frying pan

Dipping Sauce:

- 4 tablespoons nonfat Greek yogurt
- 4 tablespoons light sour cream
- A dash of parsley flakes, paprika, pepper, and sea salt

Start by washing and peeling the carrots, then grate them–measure roughly 3 cups. Dice the scallions, white and light green parts only.

In a large bowl, combine the following: grated carrots, half of the diced scallions (save the remaining for garnish), all-purpose flour (or rice flour), panko breadcrumbs (or gluten-free breadcrumbs), eggs (premix), dried parsley flakes, paprika, a dash of sea salt and black pepper, and shredded mozzarella cheese. Mix well to combine.

In a non-stick pan, add a good drizzle of olive oil and heat on medium-high to medium heat. Use more oil as needed for frying fritters.

Use a large spoon to place a dollop of the carrot mixture, about 3 tablespoons, in the pan. You can make 3 or 4 fritters at a time, depending upon the size of your pan. Cook for 1–2 minutes a side. Carefully flip using a spatula. Heat for another 1–2 minutes.

Place the carrot fritters onto a platter and add a dash of sea salt to the top.

Prepare the Dipping Sauce.

Combine the yogurt and sour cream. Mix well. Next, add a sprinkle of parsley flakes, paprika, pepper, and sea salt.

Dip the warm carrot fritters in the dipping sauce. Alternatively, dip in applesauce like a latke. These are so yummy! My kids love them.

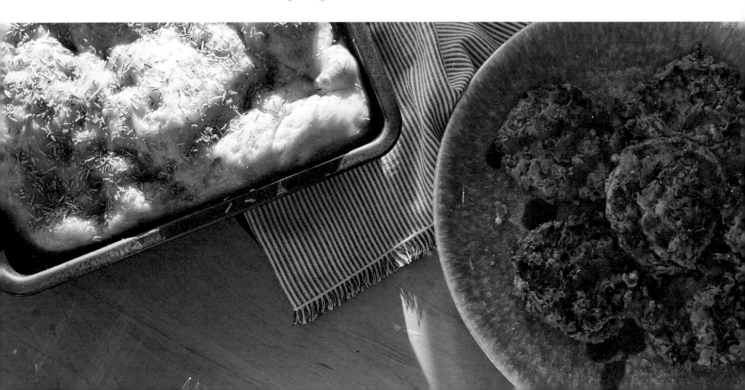

ZUCCHINI FRITTERS

INGREDIENTS:

- 2 small zucchinis (about 3 cups), grated
- ¼ cup all-purpose flour (or rice flour)
- ¼ cup grated Pecorino Romano cheese
- 1 large egg, premixed
- A dash of garlic powder
- Salt and pepper
- A good quality extra virgin olive oil
- 10-inch non-stick frying pan
- Cheesecloth

Yogurt Sauce:

- ½ cup nonfat Greek yogurt
- ½ tablespoon fresh dill, chopped
- Garlic powder, pepper, and salt (optional)

Finely grate the zucchini and strain it through a cheesecloth to get out any excess moisture. Then combine all the ingredients in a bowl and mix.

Note: Feel free to experiment with other vegetables like peppers, scallions, carrots, and more. An easy swap for all-purpose flour is rice flour to make this adaptable to a gluten-free lifestyle.

Add 1 tablespoon of olive oil to the skillet and heat on medium-high to medium.

Scoop up 1 ½ tablespoons of batter and drop 4 patties into the pan. You'll know the pan is hot enough if it sizzles. Be careful of splattering oil. Repeat adding 1 tablespoon of oil each time you fry.

Gently press down the fritters with a rubber spatula. Cook on both sides for 2 minutes until golden brown. If you like it crispier, cook longer.

Mix yogurt with a dash of garlic powder. Sprinkle with salt and pepper. Add a tiny pinch of dill and garnish the zucchini with some dill to brighten up the dish.

Serve immediately. These are best served fresh and warm.

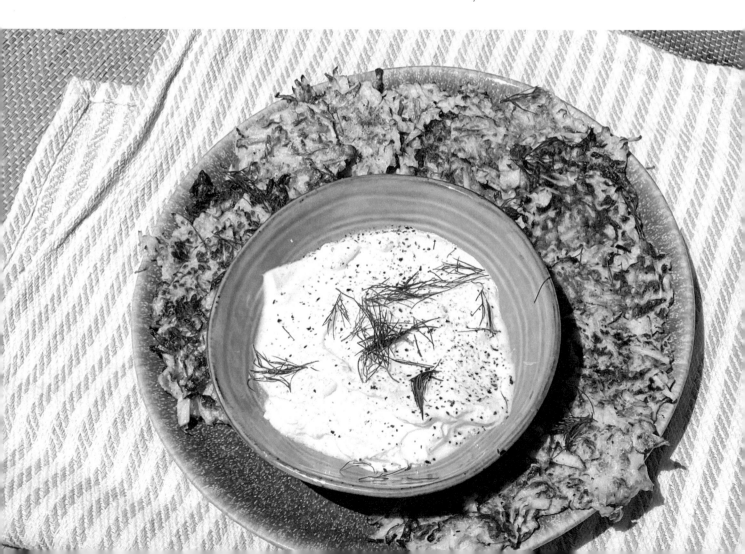

VEGETABLE PANCAKES

They are crispy around the edges from the use of rice flour and soft in the center. They are simple and so irresistible! It's a great recipe to make when you have those leftover odds and ends vegetables in your fridge. Make these for an easy dinner or Sunday morning breakfast for the family. These can be easily adapted to a gluten-free lifestyle by omitting the all-purpose flour and increasing the rice flour and cornstarch by ¼ cup each.

INGREDIENTS:

- ½ cup all-purpose flour
- ¼ cup white rice flour
- ¼ cup cornstarch
- Garlic powder to taste
- ½ teaspoon baking powder
- ¾ teaspoon fine sea salt
- ¾ cup water
- 1 large egg
- 4 cups finely chopped or grated mixed vegetables (carrots, zucchini, bell peppers, or potato)

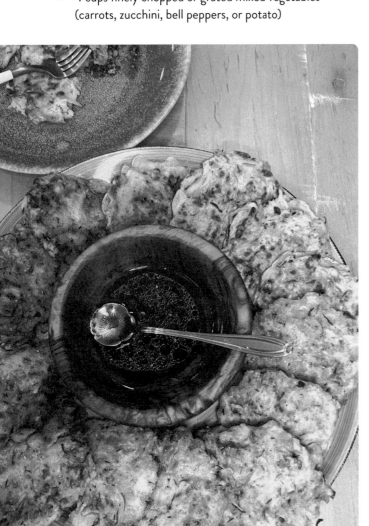

- 4 scallions, cut into 2-inch-long pieces and thinly sliced
- 2 tablespoons extra virgin olive oil (or sesame oil), plus more as needed
- 10-inch non-stick frying pan

Dipping Sauce:

- 3 tablespoons soy sauce (or gluten-free soy sauce)
- 2 teaspoons rice vinegar
- 1 teaspoon finely grated fresh ginger
- 1 teaspoon finely grated garlic
- 1 tablespoon chopped scallions
- ½ teaspoon extra virgin olive oil (or sesame oil)
- A pinch of granulated sugar

Prepare the Pancakes.

In a large bowl, whisk together all-purpose flour, rice flour, cornstarch, garlic powder, baking powder, and sea salt.

In a medium bowl, combine water and egg. Whisk the mixture into the dry ingredients until smooth. Fold in vegetables and about three-quarters of the scallions. (Save the rest for garnish.)

In a skillet over medium heat, heat 2 tablespoons of oil. Scoop ¼ cup portions of batter into the skillet, as many as will fit without touching. Flatten and fry until dark golden on the bottom, about 2–3 minutes.

Flip and continue to fry on the other side until browned, 2–3 minutes. Transfer to a paper towel-lined plate and sprinkle with a little more salt. Continue the process with the remaining batter, using more oil as needed.

Make the Dipping Sauce.

In a small bowl, stir together soy sauce, rice vinegar, ginger, garlic, scallions, olive oil, and a pinch of sugar. Sprinkle sliced scallions over the pancakes and serve with dipping sauce on the side.

MEXICAN STREET CORN ON THE COB
(Gluten Free)

SERVES 4-5

INGREDIENTS:

- 8 medium ears sweet corn, husks removed
- 1 cup light sour cream
- 1 small package cotija cheese, grated
- Gluten-free Elote Seasonings
- Salt to taste
- Chopped cilantro (optional), recommended

Boil or grill corn. If you boil the corn, drain it well. If you are grilling the corn, get a nice char on it.

> *Note: Cotija cheese is white in color, firm in texture, and has a salty flavor like feta cheese.*

In the meantime, set up 3 plates:

- *Sour cream*
- *Grated cotija cheese*
- *Diced cilantro (optional)*

Once the corn has slightly cooled and is easy to handle, roll the corn in the sour cream, then roll in grated cheese. Sprinkle Elote seasonings and diced cilantro.

Serve warm. Refrigerate any leftovers and add to a salad next day. Easy and delicious.

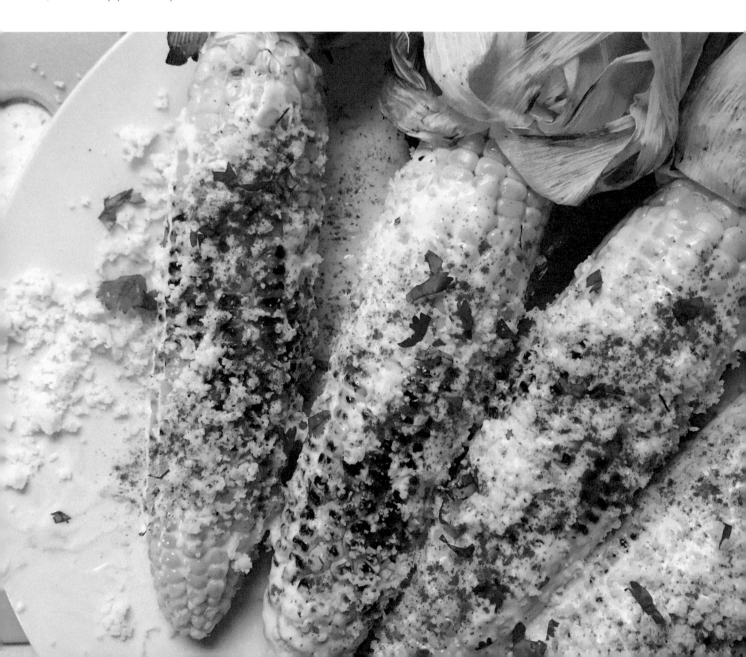

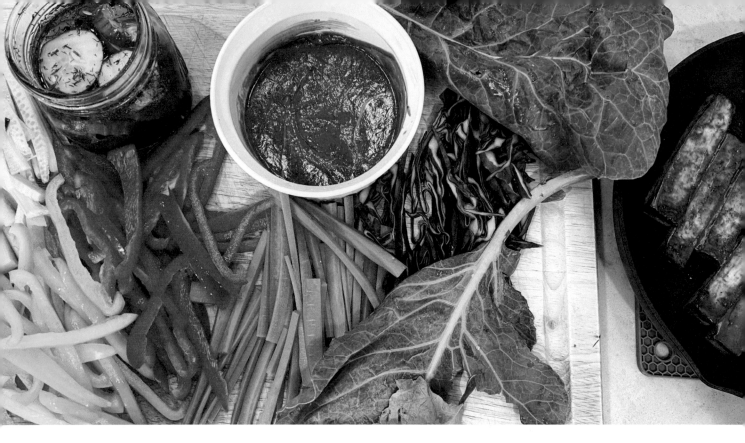

COLLARD GREEN VEGGIE WRAPS
WITH SEARED TOFU
(Gluten Free)

INGREDIENTS:

- ½ (16-ounce) package firm gluten-free tofu
- Garlic powder to taste
- ½ cup gluten-free tamari sauce
- 4 large collard green leaves plus 2 smaller ones, blanched
- ½ red pepper, thinly sliced
- ½ yellow or orange pepper, thinly sliced
- ½ English cucumber, thinly sliced
- 1 carrot, thinly sliced
- ½ cup chopped red cabbage
- Homemade pickles (recipe follows)
- Extra virgin olive oil
- Pastry brush
- Small frying pan
- Large, wide pot

Tahini-Tamari Dipping Sauce:

- ⅓ cup tahini
- ¼ cup gluten-free tamari sauce
- 1 teaspoon gluten-free chili garlic sauce
- Water to loosen

Homemade Pickles:

- 1 small English cucumber (from your garden)
- Crinkle cutter
- Distilled White vinegar
- Water
- Whole peppercorns
- Black pepper and table salt
- Dried dill
- Green goddess dry herbs (optional)
- 8-ounce jar with tight-fitting lid

First, prepare the pickles in advance. Let them soak overnight.

Make the Homemade Pickles.

Using the crinkle cutter, cut thin circles widthwise (or you can cut them thicker as seen in photo). Add the cucumbers to the jar. Next, add equal parts vinegar and water and a generous amount of the following seasonings: peppercorns, black pepper, salt, dried dill, and the green goddess dry herb blend. Let this soak overnight.

Money saving tip: I will save store-bought pickle jars or other jars, clean thoroughly in the dishwasher, and reuse them for homemade pickles, onions, salad dressing, pesto, or jams.

Start by drying the block of tofu. Cut slices widthwise, about ¾-inch wide. Then cut each slice in half to make 8 long lengthwise pieces and sprinkle with garlic powder for flavor. Soak the pieces in tamari sauce for 15 minutes. Be sure to pour some over the top using a spoon.

Next, add a drizzle of oil to the pan and sear the tofu on each side for about 4 minutes until nicely charred. Set aside to slightly cool.

Blanch each collard green leaf in simmering water for 20 seconds, until bright green and slightly tender. Pat dry. Next, trim back the spine of each leaf, so the leaf lays as flat as possible. You should be able to bend the leaf without it cracking.

Chef's tip: Cutting toward the stem end will give you more control, going the other way you may accidentally cut into the leaf, making a hole. If you do, you can use the tiny collard greens to patch the hole.

Cut the peppers, cucumbers, carrots, and cabbage as thin as possible into matchstick or julienne vegetables—a good chef's knife is very important here. Keep the vegetables separated into individual piles. Chop some homemade pickles or you can leave them whole and add them into the wraps.

Use any crunchy vegetables you have on hand: carrots, peppers, radishes, cucumbers, zucchini, scallions, or beets. Also, some add in ideas for more crunch: microgreens, fresh parsley, fresh dill, or homemade Pickled Red Onions (page 56). For more protein ideas: cooked steak or chicken in lieu of tofu.

Prepare the Tahini-Tamari Dipping Sauce.

Combine the tahini, tamari, and chili garlic sauce, and whisk. Add water to slightly loosen. Using a pastry brush, brush onto the tamari-seared tofu for added flavor.

Lay the leaf flat onto a cutting board. At the top of the leaf, add the tofu and julienne veggies, tuck in left side, then right side, and start to roll. Smear on a little bit of the sauce at the end and do the final tuck. Cut in half, slip in some pickles, and enjoy!

Alternative sauce idea: I have used a Tahini-Lemon Yogurt Sauce with fresh dill and garlic powder, equally good!

Nutrition tip: A good rule of thumb is to have a wide variety of vegetables and fruit: eat the rainbow. This way you ensure you are getting an array of vitamins and minerals to support a healthy lifestyle.

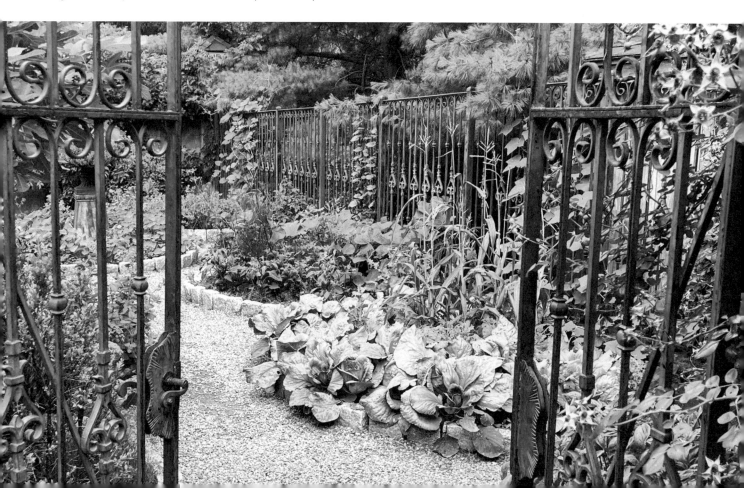

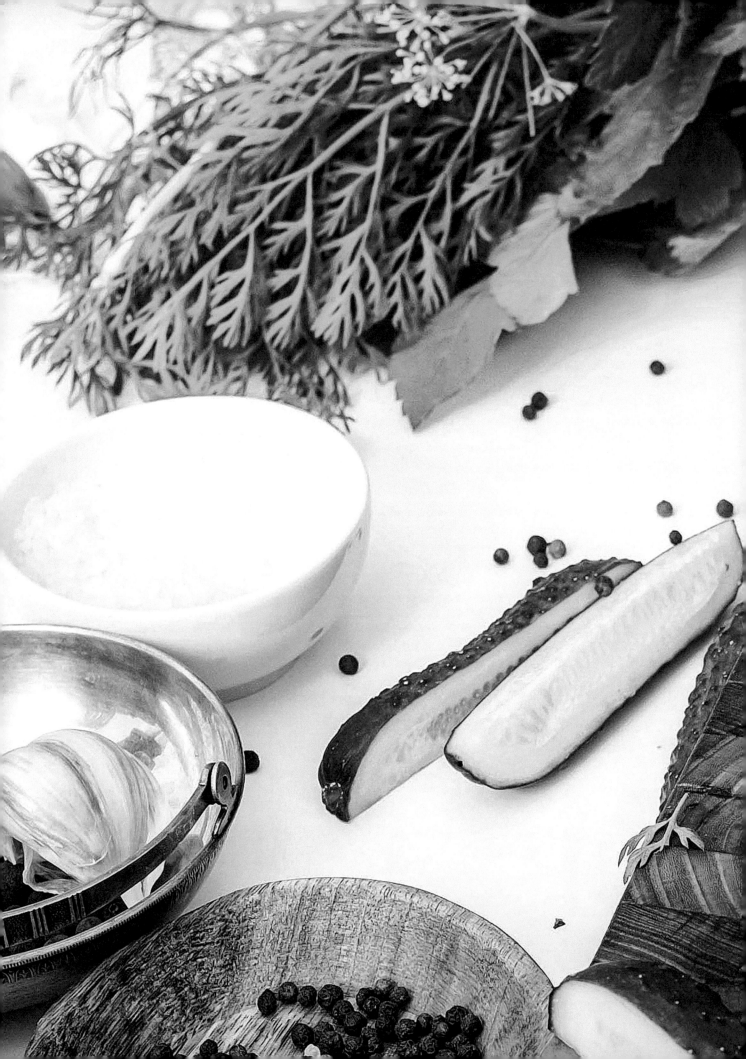

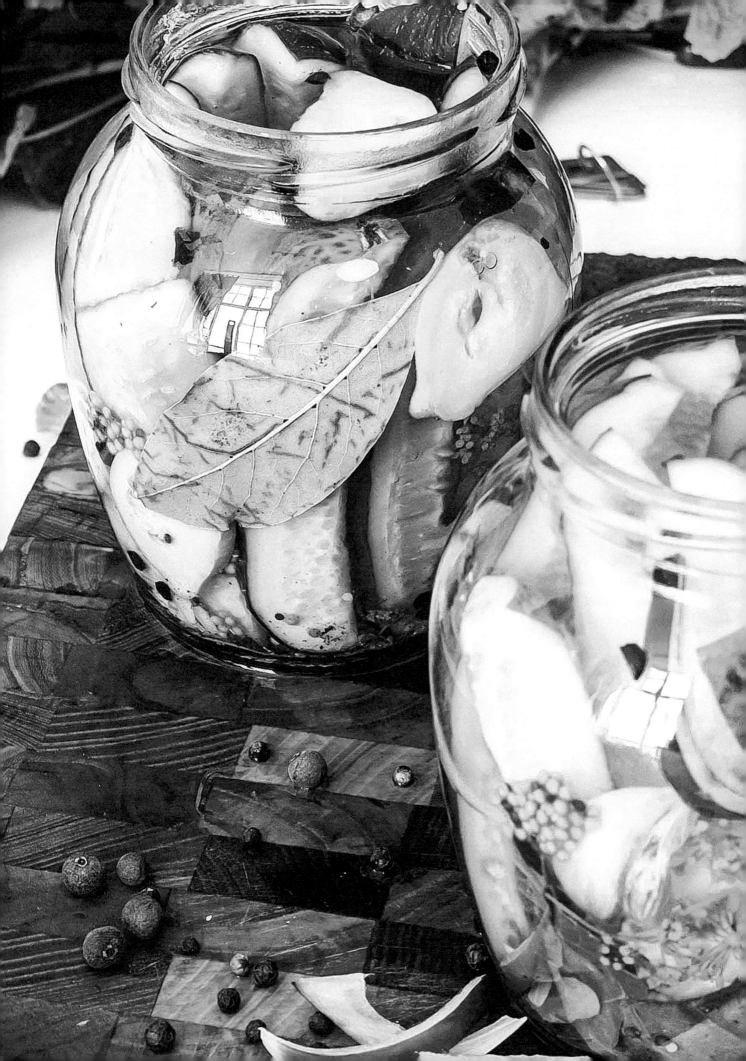

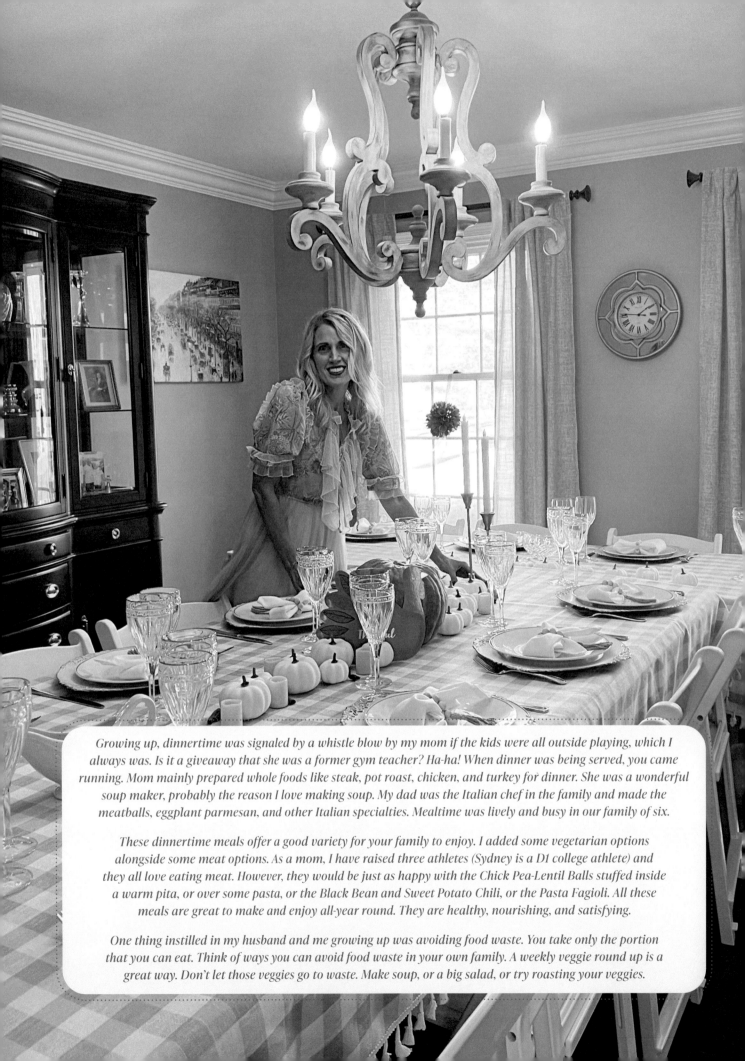

Growing up, dinnertime was signaled by a whistle blow by my mom if the kids were all outside playing, which I always was. Is it a giveaway that she was a former gym teacher? Ha-ha! When dinner was being served, you came running. Mom mainly prepared whole foods like steak, pot roast, chicken, and turkey for dinner. She was a wonderful soup maker, probably the reason I love making soup. My dad was the Italian chef in the family and made the meatballs, eggplant parmesan, and other Italian specialties. Mealtime was lively and busy in our family of six.

These dinnertime meals offer a good variety for your family to enjoy. I added some vegetarian options alongside some meat options. As a mom, I have raised three athletes (Sydney is a D1 college athlete) and they all love eating meat. However, they would be just as happy with the Chick Pea-Lentil Balls stuffed inside a warm pita, or over some pasta, or the Black Bean and Sweet Potato Chili, or the Pasta Fagioli. All these meals are great to make and enjoy all-year round. They are healthy, nourishing, and satisfying.

One thing instilled in my husband and me growing up was avoiding food waste. You take only the portion that you can eat. Think of ways you can avoid food waste in your own family. A weekly veggie round up is a great way. Don't let those veggies go to waste. Make soup, or a big salad, or try roasting your veggies.

DINNERTIME

ASIAN-INSPIRED TURKEY MEATBALLS
WITH SOBA NOODLES

PASTA FAGIOLI

CHICK PEA-LENTIL BALLS
(Gluten Free)

BEEF BOURGUIGNON
(Gluten Free)

BLACK BEAN AND SWEET POTATO CHILI
(Gluten Free)

BREADED CHICKEN CUTLETS
WITH PROSCIUTTO AND GOAT CHEESE

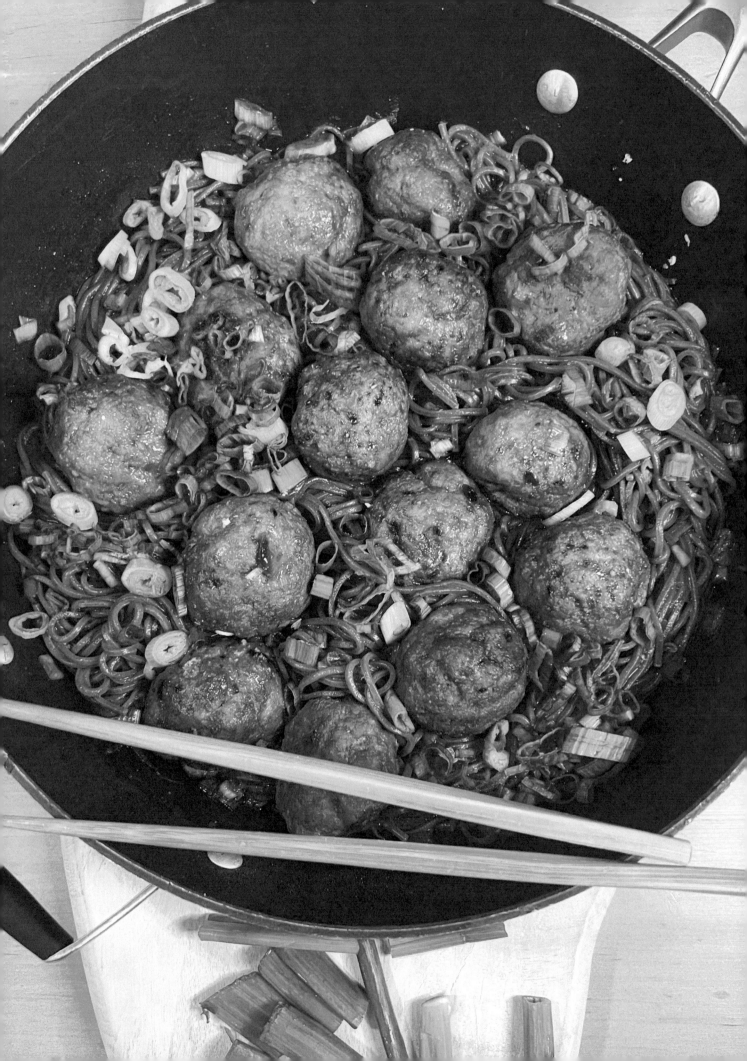

ASIAN-INSPIRED TURKEY MEATBALLS
WITH SOBA NOODLES

INGREDIENTS:

- 1 ½ lbs. ground turkey, 85-90% lean
- ½ cup cornflake breadcrumbs (or gluten-free breadcrumbs)
- 3–4 tablespoon soy sauce (or gluten-free soy sauce)
- Garlic powder to taste
- A tiny sprinkle of ground ginger
- Salt
- Red chili flakes
- Medium-sized non-stick frying pan
- Chopsticks for eating
- Soba noodles (made from buckwheat)

Asian-Inspired Sauce:

- ⅓ cup tamari (or soy sauce) (or gluten-free tamari or soy sauce)
- 2 tablespoon extra virgin olive oil (or sesame oil)
- 1 tablespoon rice vinegar
- 1 teaspoon honey
- Freshly grated ginger (about 1 tablespoon or more)
- ¼ cup diced scallions
- ¼ cup water (or more)
- 6 more scallion stalks for topping dish, thinly sliced

For a vegetarian spin on this dish, omit the turkey meatballs and instead use the recipe for seared tofu from the Collard Green Veggie Wrap (page 76). Add it to the soba noodles in lieu of the turkey meatballs. Just don't over toss the tofu with the soba noodles, as it is delicate. Either way, these are *soba* good. Ha-ha!

Preheat the oven to 375 degrees.

In a large bowl, mix the ground turkey, breadcrumbs, soy sauce, garlic powder, ginger, salt, and red chili flakes. You will make about 14 meatballs. Place them onto a parchment-lined baking sheet.

Bake for 35–40 minutes until browned on bottom and no longer pink.

While the meatballs are cooking, prepare the sauce. In the medium-sized non-stick skillet, add the tamari, olive oil, rice vinegar, honey, freshly grated ginger, 1 tablespoon or more of diced scallions, and about ¼ cup of water. Heat on medium-low heat. Reserve some scallions for topping.

While the sauce is cooking and the meatballs are close to being done, prepare the soba noodles. Always check the ingredient label for the presence of wheat.

Despite the name *buckwheat*, there are brands that are gluten free. If you can't find those, try to find sticky noodles, like rice noodles, as an alternative, which are equally delicious!

I cooked 5 stacks of soba noodles, so about 5 portions for this meal. You must boil the noodles; they have a quick cooking time, about 5 minutes. Always follow package directions. Then, thoroughly rinse the noodles, unlike what you would do with pasta.

Add the cooked meatballs to the sauce and allow them to simmer on low heat for about 10 minutes to meld the flavors. Be sure the meatballs have reached the safe internal temperature. You can reference foodsafety.gov for a list of safe internal temperatures.

Once the soba noodles are drained, transfer the meatballs to a bowl. Add the soba noodles to the pan and mix with the sauce. Transfer the meatballs back into the pan with the noodles and top with thinly sliced scallions, or if you made tofu, top the noodles with tofu and scallions.

This is so good. Enjoy! Serve with chopsticks.

PASTA FAGIOLI

SERVES 6

This Pasta Fagioli recipe is like the traditional pasta fagioli recipe made in Italy. I decided to add it to the Dinnertime chapter of my book, because although it's more like a soup, it's very hearty. The textures and flavors in this soup are so complex and delicious. It will keep you and your family coming back for more. It's a great option for those colder days when you want something warm and nourishing. It's also easy to pull together on those busy days and use leftover veggies in the fridge to avoid food waste. It is also a budget-friendly meal.

INGREDIENTS:

- 2 (15.5-ounce) cans cannellini beans, rinsed and drained
- 3 large carrots, peeled and diced
- 2 celery stalks, peeled and diced
- 1 small onion, diced (or 1 leek)
- 1 tablespoon salted butter (or rendered pancetta fat)
- 3 cloves garlic, diced (about 1 tablespoon)
- 2 (32-ounce) containers chicken (or vegetable stock)
- 2 (14.5-ounce) cans fire-roasted tomatoes (or 1 (28-ounce) can San Marzano whole peeled tomatoes)
- 2–3 fresh thyme sprigs
- 3 bay leaves
- 1–2 teaspoons granulated sugar (optional)
- Salt and pepper to taste
- Fresh parsley, chopped
- A good quality extra virgin olive oil
- Freshly grated Parmigiano-Reggiano cheese for serving
- 1 ½ cups cooked Ditalini pasta (or gluten-free pasta)
- Large pot with tight-fitting lid
- Potato masher

Rinse the beans in a colander and drain. Set them aside.

Dice the carrots, celery, and onion. This should measure roughly 4 cups of vegetables for this recipe. Add a drizzle of oil to a pot along with the butter (or rendered pancetta fat). Add the vegetables and garlic and lightly salt. Heat on medium for 8 minutes.

Note: If you would like to add some chopped pancetta, you may do so along with the vegetables. That will give an extra layer of flavor to this already delicious dish.

Take the sautéed vegetables out of the pot and add them to a large metal bowl. Add 1 container of stock (reserve the other) to the pot along with half of the beans. Bring it to a boil for a few minutes, then lower to simmer. This is especially important if the beans are hard. Use a potato masher to mash the beans. This will thicken the broth.

Next, add the vegetables (and pancetta if you added it)

back into the pot along with remaining beans, fire roasted tomatoes, 2 fresh thyme springs, and bay leaves. Sugar, salt, and pepper may be added to taste. Add a large handful of chopped parsley, or as much or as little as you like.

Note: If you are using the San Marzano whole peeled tomatoes instead of the fire-roasted tomatoes, rinse out the seeds, crush with your hands, and add to the soup.

Allow this to simmer. In the meantime, prepare the pasta. Once it's cooked, add 1 ½ cups to the soup.

Note: The pasta will become soggy over time and absorb most of the broth, so if you prefer, add the pasta to individual servings. Otherwise, you'll need at least half of a container more of stock, so keep it on hand.

Some other variations are to use kidney beans, add in other veggies like zucchini and potatoes. This is a great meal to adapt based on what's in the fridge and what's in season.

Taste the soup after 45 minutes or so. This is an important element of cooking. Or better yet, dip a chunk of bread into it. Adjust seasonings to your liking. Keep on a low simmer.

Serve with shaved Parmigiano-Reggiano cheese and a chunk of crusty Italian bread. As a garnish add fresh chopped parsley. Expect this meal to disappear fast. Call the family: soups on!

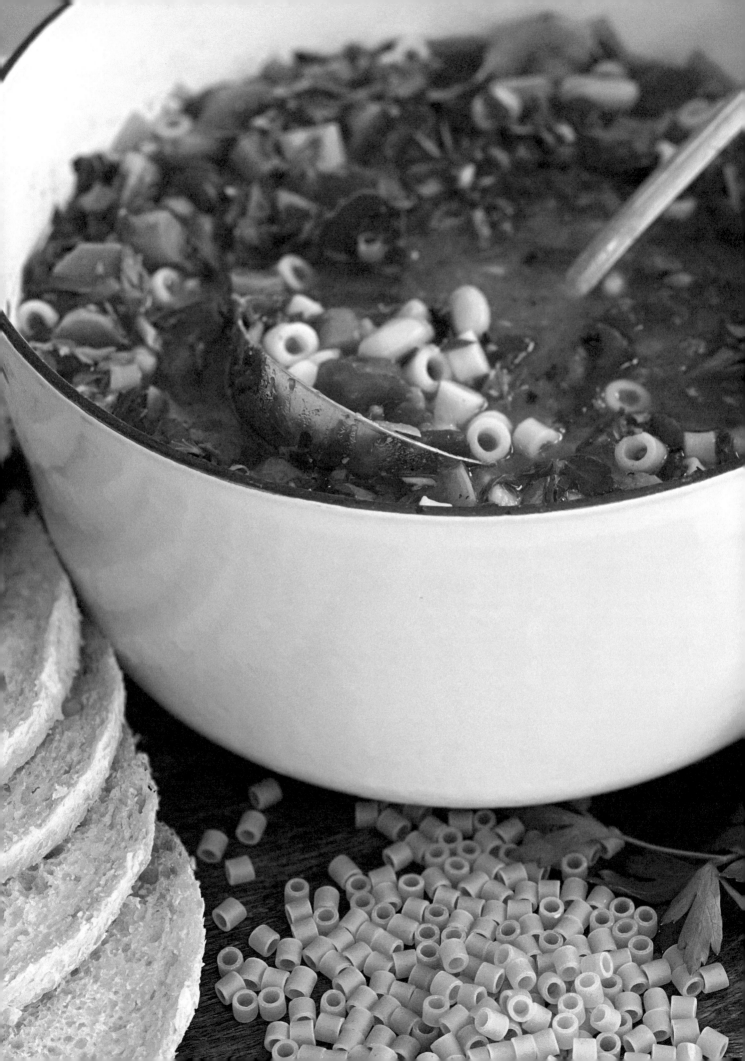

CHICK PEA-LENTIL BALLS
(Gluten Free)

INGREDIENTS:

- 2 cups chick peas, rinsed and drained (about 1 large can)
- 1 ½ cups cooked brown lentils, store-bought
- ½ onion, finely diced (or onion powder)
- 2 tablespoons flax meal
- ¼ teaspoon garlic powder (or more)
- 2 tablespoons parsley flakes (or 1 tablespoon fresh parsley, or chives)
- 1 large egg
- 2 tablespoons rice flour (or all-purpose flour)
- Black pepper and ground sea salt
- Red chili flakes (optional)
- A good quality extra virgin olive oil
- High-speed blender
- Medium-sized non-stick frying pan
- Non-stick cooking spray

Preheat the oven to 350 degrees.

In the high-speed blender, combine the chick peas, cooked lentils, and onions. Pulse until the mixture is well combined and chunky, not smooth like hummus.

Note: I used half of a 16-ounce package of precooked brown lentils, this saved a significant amount of time. If you can find them precooked, use them. Otherwise, rinse dry lentils. Fill a pot halfway with water and add dry lentils. Bring to a boil, then simmer for 20–30 minutes until softened. Allow them to cool before adding the lentils to the blender.

Place the mixture into a medium-sized bowl. Add the onion, flax meal, garlic powder, parsley, salt, and pepper. Before you add the flour and egg, taste the mixture to be sure the flavors are to your liking. You might like more garlic powder or even some spice like red chili flakes. Last, add in a pre-mixed egg and the flour. Mix until everything forms together.

Next, scoop up about 2 heaping tablespoons of the mixture. Make a ball and place onto a parchment-lined baking sheet. Spray the balls with non-stick cooking spray.

Place in the oven to bake for 25 minutes, turn halfway through. Spray again once you turn them.

For an extra crispy ball (recommended):

In a non-stick frying pan, add a few tablespoons of olive oil and heat on low. Then add the balls. Cook until golden brown and crispy.

Serve with tahini or tzatziki. Smash balls between 2 pieces of warmed pita to make a sandwich. This is a nutritious and delicious meal paired with my Mezze Platter (page 37).

Alternatively, pair these with a red sauce mixed with tahini, which is reminiscent of a vodka sauce but healthier. Add some basil ribbons.

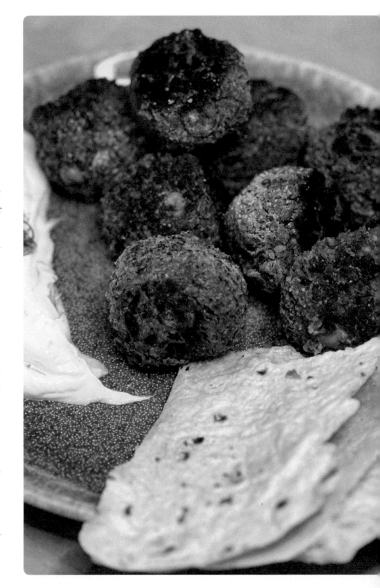

BEEF BOURGUIGNON
(Gluten Free)

Beef Bourguignon is a French beef stew braised with a dry red wine. The key to a wonderful bourguignon is layers of flavor, and of course, a lot of red wine. The potatoes are typically added in at the end of the cooking process, so feel free to boil them and cook separately. My husband loves beef stew with potatoes. In this recipe, we will be braising the meat along with the diced potatoes.

INGREDIENTS:

- 2 lbs. chuck beef, cut into 1 ½-inch chunks
- 3 tablespoons cornstarch
- ½ large leek, cut in half lengthwise, diced
- 2 celery stalks, peeled and diced
- 3 large carrots, peeled and thinly cut widthwise
- 1 small bag frozen white pearl onions, cooked and drained (or 1 medium onion, sliced)
- A good quality extra virgin olive oil
- Sea salt and black pepper to taste
- 1 cup red wine (cabernet or pinot noir)
- ½ container beef stock (about 2 ½ cups)
- 1–2 tablespoon GravyMaster®
- Thyme sprigs
- 3–4 Russet potatoes, peeled and cut into 1-inch chunks (about 5 cups, or baby Dutch yellow potatoes cut in half)
- 3–4 bay leaves
- 1–2 tablespoons tomato paste (optional)
- Wide-mouthed, medium-sized Dutch oven, or ceramic coated cast-iron skillet with a tight-fitting lid

Preheat the oven to 325 degrees. The pan will go in the middle of the oven, so prepare the rack so it fits with the lid.

Pat the beef dry with a paper towel. It should have a fair amount of marbling, but you can cut off any excess fat. Lightly salt the meat and add it to a large plastic bag. Add the cornstarch, seal the bag, and shake it to fully coat the beef. Alternatively, you may use all-purpose flour. I used cornstarch as a gluten free alternative.

Cut the leeks in half lengthwise and dice (widthwise). Then add them to a bowl filled with water. Peel and dice the celery and add it to the bowl. Both tend to have a fair amount of dirt. Let them soak, then drain, rinse, and drain again.

In the meantime, peel and cut the carrots thinly widthwise. Heat the pearl onions according to bag directions and drain out any excess liquid. Tie together 6 thyme sprigs with kitchen string.

Note: The pearl onions should not have any other added ingredients, otherwise, it will impact the flavor of this dish.

Drizzle a little olive oil in the bottom of the pan, add the leeks, celery, carrots, and pearl onions and allow this to heat for about 6 minutes on medium heat. Add a pinch of salt and pepper. Then take the vegetables out of the pan and add to a bowl.

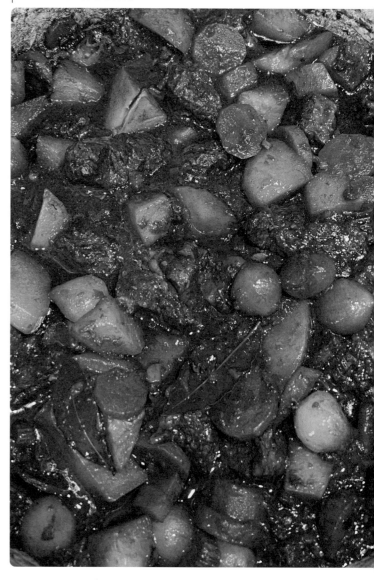

Optional step: Add a tablespoon of tomato paste to the vegetables and mix.

Add a good drizzle of olive oil to the pan and allow it to heat. Then add the cornstarch-coated beef. Do not overcrowd the pan. You want to brown the beef on all sides, so keep turning. Do it in batches if necessary. Keep the heat on medium. If the meat sticks, add more olive oil. The meat will not be fully cooked, just browned.

Next, take the meat out and transfer to a bowl. Off the heat, add the red wine and beef stock. Place it back onto the burner and bring it to a boil for a minute. Then reduce heat to simmer and scrape up all the bits with a flat-edged wooden spoon.

Note: Wine is flammable, deglaze the pan off the heat.

Add the vegetables and beef back into the pan along with 2 tablespoons of Gravy Master®. Let this simmer for 5 minutes. Toss in the bundled thyme sprigs. Toss in the diced potatoes. The liquid should just about cover the stew. You can add more stock, if necessary, about ½ cup. Add the bay leaves.

Note: I have seen recipes where you cook the meat first and then cook the vegetables, but in those cases, you do not add the flour/cornstarch to the meat. You can do it that way, but then add the cornstarch to the liquid (wine/ beef stock) and whisk it until no lumps remain. You want to create a thick gravy.

Place the lid on the pan and place in the oven to braise for 2 hours. Check halfway through and stir.

Harvest tip: Leeks are a spring vegetable, so you will see them make an appearance in April at your local farmer's market. Feel free to use fresh pearl onions if you can find them at the local farmer's market. Harvest season for pearl onions is summer to early fall. Carrots are summer to late fall.

Nutrition tip: Increasing the nutritional profile of your food is as simple as buying local area produce from the farmer's markets and local farm stands. As produce travels, it loses its nutritional profile. That's why farm-to-table cooking is always best.

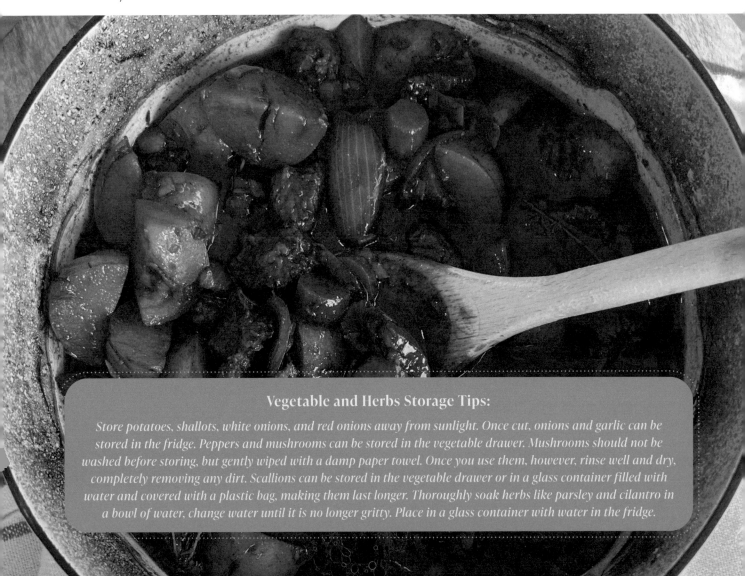

Vegetable and Herbs Storage Tips:

Store potatoes, shallots, white onions, and red onions away from sunlight. Once cut, onions and garlic can be stored in the fridge. Peppers and mushrooms can be stored in the vegetable drawer. Mushrooms should not be washed before storing, but gently wiped with a damp paper towel. Once you use them, however, rinse well and dry, completely removing any dirt. Scallions can be stored in the vegetable drawer or in a glass container filled with water and covered with a plastic bag, making them last longer. Thoroughly soak herbs like parsley and cilantro in a bowl of water, change water until it is no longer gritty. Place in a glass container with water in the fridge.

BLACK BEAN AND SWEET POTATO CHILI
(Gluten Free)

INGREDIENTS:

- 2 (29-ounce) cans black beans, rinsed and drained
- 1 small red pepper, seeded and diced
- 1 small orange pepper, seeded and diced
- 1 small yellow pepper, seeded and diced
- 1 yellow onion, diced
- 1 large sweet potato, peeled and diced
- 1 cup sliced baby bella mushrooms (or shitake mushrooms)
- 1 small container chicken stock (or vegetable broth), use ¾ of container
- ½ cup red wine, pinot noir
- Splash of gluten-free summer ale
- 1 (26-ounce) jar prepared tomato sauce (or crushed tomato sauce)
- 2–3 cloves garlic, whole
- 3 tablespoons gluten free hot sauce
- 2 teaspoons chili powder
- 1 lime, squeezed
- 2–3 bay leaves
- Black pepper, ground sea salt, red chili flakes, and paprika to taste
- 1 can of adobe peppers (optional)
- A good quality extra virgin olive oil
- Large pot with tight-fitting lid
- Garnish: red onion, scallions, pepper jack cheese (shredded), and sour cream

Rinse and drain the black beans, then set those aside. Cut the tops off the peppers, rinse and remove all seeds and pulp, then dice the peppers and onion.

Fun facts: Green peppers are harvested early, before they have a chance to turn yellow, orange, and finally red.

Drizzle the olive oil in a large pot. Add the diced onion and peppers along with a good sprinkle of ground sea salt and a few good sprinkles of red chili flakes. Let it simmer for 10 minutes on low heat to soften.

Note: You may adapt this recipe and add carrots in lieu of peppers. In this case, add 4 large carrots. These pair well with sweet potatoes. You may also swap out the sweet potatoes for some roasted pumpkin.

In the meantime, peel the sweet potato and dice it into

bite-sized pieces. Use a good chef's knife to dice the potato. Add it to the pot with peppers and onions. Slice the mushrooms and add those to the pan. Add a drizzle more of olive oil and a good sprinkle of black pepper. Allow this to cook for 8 minutes to soften the sweet potatoes and partially cook the mushrooms.

Next, add the black beans to the pot along with ¾ of the container of chicken stock (reserve the rest), wine, splash beer, jarred sauce, garlic, hot sauce, chili powder, lime juice, bay leaves, more black pepper, and a few dashes of paprika.

Mix the chili to incorporate the ingredients. Keep on low heat for 2 hours or longer. The chili will appear liquidy at first, but most of the liquid will evaporate after roughly 2 hours.

Garnish with red onion, chopped scallions, cheese, and a dollop of sour cream. Serve with homemade gluten-free bread (or Italian bread).

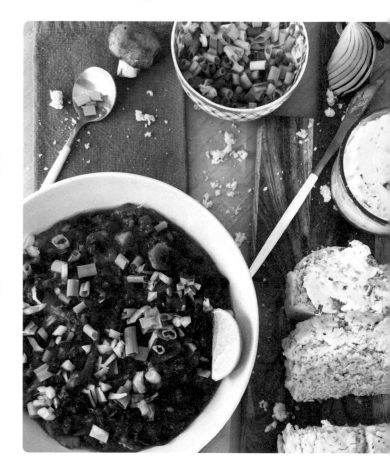

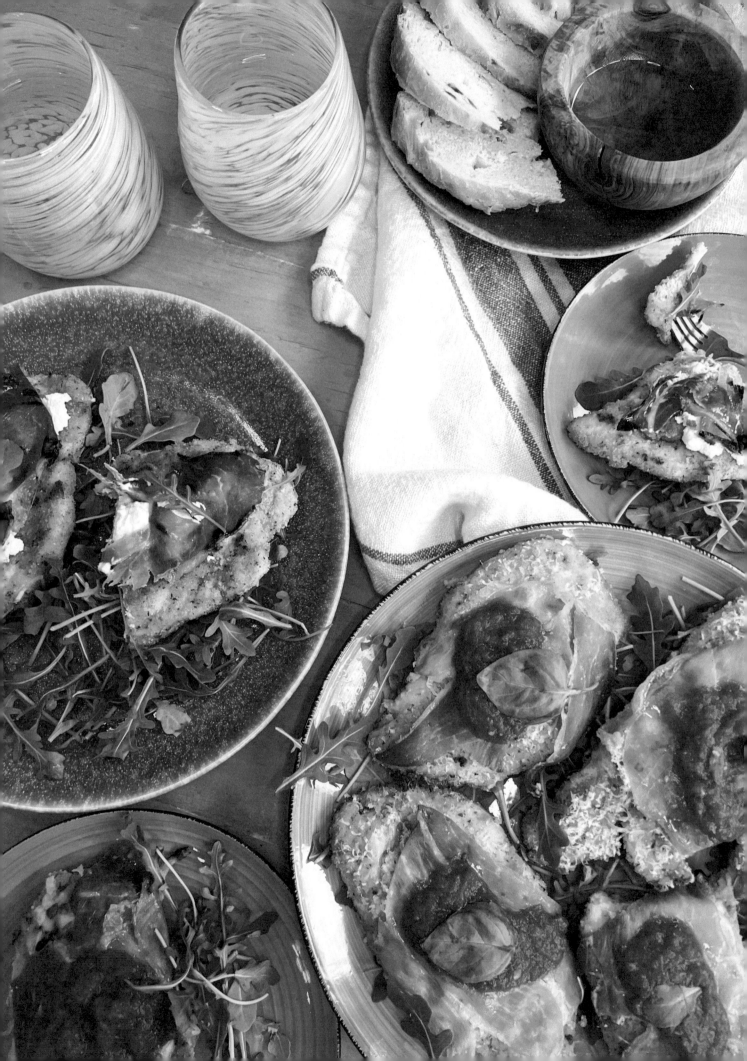

BREADED CHICKEN CUTLETS
WITH PROSCIUTTO AND GOAT CHEESE

INGREDIENTS:

- 4 large chicken breast cutlets, halved (about 3 lbs.; makes 8 cutlets)
- 1 cup Italian seasoned breadcrumbs (or gluten free breadcrumbs)
- ¼ cup panko breadcrumbs (or gluten free panko breadcrumbs)
- ¼ cup grated Parmigiano-Reggiano (or parmesan) cheese
- 1 cup all-purpose flour (or cornstarch)
- 1 cup low-fat milk or 2–3 eggs
- 1 (4-ounce) package Prosciutto di Parma slices (about 8 slices)
- 1 (5-ounce) package Chèvre cheese (goat cheese)
- Honey
- A good quality extra virgin olive oil
- Garlic powder and sea salt to taste
- 1 small box arugula
- Balsamic Glaze (optional)

Preheat the oven to 425 degrees.

> *Fun fact: Parmigiano-Reggiano is made in Italy. Parmesan cheese is made in America. They will have slightly different tastes. Prosciutto Di Parma is a good quality prosciutto from Italy as well, use that for this recipe.*

Prepare 2 baking sheets with parchment paper.

Cut the chicken cutlets in half lengthwise, creating 8 cutlets. Add 2 cutlets at a time to a large plastic bag and pound the cutlets out about ¾-inch thickness. Do this on a cutting board that is dishwasher safe.

In a bowl, combine the Italian-seasoned breadcrumbs with the panko breadcrumbs and cheese and mix. Season with garlic powder and salt.

Set up three bowls:

- *Flour*
- *Milk (or egg)*
- *Breadcrumbs*

Dredge the cutlets in flour, milk (or premixed egg), then breadcrumbs. Place onto the parchment-lined baking sheet. Spray with non-stick cooking spray.

Bake the cutlets for 15 minutes, then flip and spray again. Bake an additional 15 minutes until meat is cooked through and reaches safe internal temperature. If you wish to have the outside crispier, add a drizzle of oil to a non-stick frying pan and sauté for 2 minutes a side until crispy and golden brown.

In the meantime, cut the prosciutto slices in half lengthwise. Once the chicken is done, crumble on some goat cheese on the top of each cutlet, then add the halved slices. Drizzle with honey and bake until the prosciutto gets crispy, about 4–5 minutes.

Add the cutlets onto a bed of arugula and drizzle on some balsamic glaze. There is a recipe for Balsamic Glaze (page 57). You can serve the cutlets with a vegetable side and some homemade Italian bread (or gluten-free bread) for a light dinner. As an alternative idea, you may add parmesan cheese to the tops of the cutlets, then top with prosciutto. Once heated, add tomato sauce, as seen in the photo.

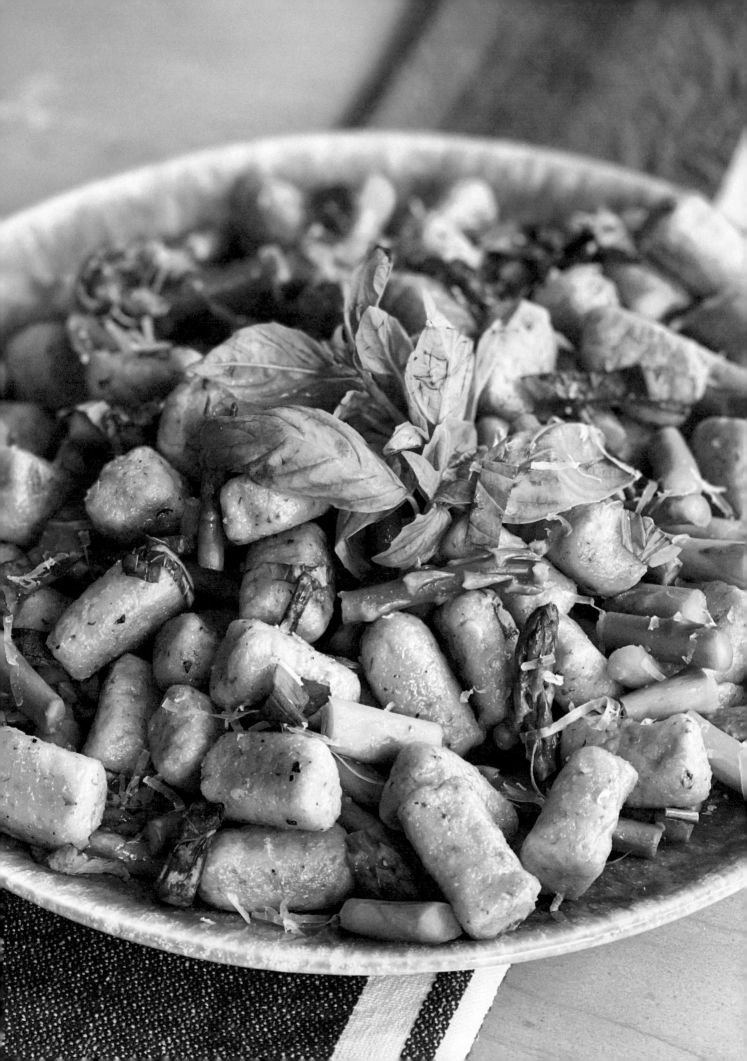

PASTA, POTATO DUMPLINGS, AND SAUCES

END OF SUMMER HARVEST GREEN-RED TOMATO SAUCE
(Gluten Free)

SWEET POTATO GNOCCHI
(Gluten Free)

POTATO DUMPLINGS

MUSHROOM RAGU WITH PAPPARDELLE

RED LENTIL BOLOGNESE
WITH CREAMY PARMESAN POLENTA
(Gluten Free)

SPAGHETTI ALLA NERANO

PESTO PENNE PASTA

END OF SUMMER HARVEST GREEN-RED TOMATO SAUCE

*Allow 5 hours to simmer

INGREDIENTS:

- 6 medium-sized green tomatoes
- 2 large red beefsteak tomatoes
- 4 cups water
- 1 medium-sized onion, diced
- 3–4 garlic cloves, thinly sliced
- 4 San Marzano canned whole peeled tomatoes plus 3 tablespoons liquid
- 5 tablespoons extra virgin olive oil
- ¼ teaspoon dried oregano
- ¾ teaspoon sea salt
- ¼ teaspoon black pepper
- 2–3 dried bay leaves
- A pinch of sugar
- 1 tablespoon tomato paste (optional)
- Food mill
- High-speed blender
- Large pot with lid
- Tongs

Step One: With a paring knife make an X at the bottom of the tomatoes, this will make it easy to peel away the skin once simmered. Place the tomatoes in the pot with 4 cups of water and 3 tablespoons of olive oil (reserve the rest). Toss in half the diced onions (reserve the remaining onions). Simmer on medium-low heat until softened and skin starts to peel away, about 10-15 minutes.

Step Two: Use the tongs to take out the tomatoes, then once cool enough to handle, pull off the skin and core them. This means you cut out the part that the tomato used to attach to the stem. It doesn't have to be perfect. Any leftover skin will be caught by the food mill. Cut the tomatoes in half and scoop out seeds (or rinse them).

Step Three: Add the tomatoes and onions to the food mill. First, break them up with your hands. Then crank the handle and allow the sauce to drop into another bowl, catching all the seeds and any skin you missed in the top part of the food mill. Be sure to scrape the bottom of the food mill, as some of the sauce will be stuck. Add that to the liquid in the bowl.

Step Four: In the pot, add the thinly sliced garlic with 2 tablespoons (or more) of olive oil. Keep the heat on low and cook about 4 minutes. Do not brown. Add the remaining diced onions to the pan with the garlic (this is in addition to the onions you boiled with the tomatoes.)

Step Five: Add the strained liquid back into the pot with the garlic. Rinse 4–5 canned San Marzano tomatoes to get out the seeds. Add them to the blender with 3 tablespoons of the liquid from the can and blend. Add this to the pot along with the liquid.

Step Six: Season the mixture with oregano, salt, pepper, and a pinch of sugar. Add a bay leaf as well. The bay leaf always flavors the sauce nicely. I think the bay leaf was the secret to my Grandma's tomato sauce, a taste I have yet to replicate. In my cookbook, *Food That Will Gather Your Family*, there is a delicious Rustic Tomato Sauce Recipe, which is slightly different than this one.

Step Seven: The sauce will be very liquidy so allow it to simmer for about 4–5 hours. If you are pressed for time, you may add 2 tablespoons (or more) of tomato paste to thicken the sauce. Taste it as you go, adjusting the seasonings to your liking.

Step Eight: After about 4–5 hours, sauce will be reduced to half, thickened, and ready to use. It is incredibly delicious!

You may think August is the end of gardening season and that things are starting to wind down, but August harvest is plentiful. You will reap the rewards from all the hard work you did in the spring and early summer. Tomatoes, corn, zucchini, cucumbers, eggplant, and even some apples will be in abundance and ready to be picked. And although most of us don't plant corn in our garden, it will be popping up in local farmer's markets. The corn is ready to eat when the juice from the corn is milky rather than clear. Tomatoes can be picked when they are green or red. Pick them as you use them for different recipes, like this delicious sauce. Zucchini and cucumbers must be picked every couple of days. Pick eggplants when they are a deep blackish color and shiny.

SWEET POTATO GNOCCHI
(Gluten Free)

INGREDIENTS:

- 3–4 medium organic sweet potatoes (roughly 2 ⅔ cups packed)
- ¼ cup freshly grated Pecorino Romano cheese
- Sea salt and cracked black pepper
- A pinch of nutmeg
- 1 jumbo egg yolk
- 1 ½ cups plus 1 tablespoon (or more) King Arthurs Baking Company's Gluten-Free Measure for Measure Flour, spooned and leveled
- Wood pastry board
- Pastry scraper (or vegetable chopper)
- Potato ricer (optional, but recommended)
- Fork (or gnocchi board)
- Excess gluten-free flour for wood pastry board
- Large pot to boil gnocchi
- Spider strainer

Step One: Scrub the potatoes with a vegetable scrubber. Pierce each potato with a fork and cook them in the microwave until fork tender. Alternatively, pierce the potatoes and bake them in the oven for about 1 hour and 15 minutes (or longer) at 425 degrees. You'll want to work with the potatoes while hot, so get out as much steam as possible. Use an oven mitt to handle.

Step Two: Place the potatoes onto the wood pastry board. Hold the potato with a fork, insert a butter knife under the skin, and gently move the knife all around the potato to remove the skin. It should slide right off. Discard the potato skin. Measure roughly 2 ⅔ cups packed sweet potato and set it aside.

Step Three: Use a vegetable chopper to coarsely chop the potatoes into fine bits. This lets out all the steam. You can also use a potato ricer if you have one. Once the potato is finely chopped, add the Pecorino Romano

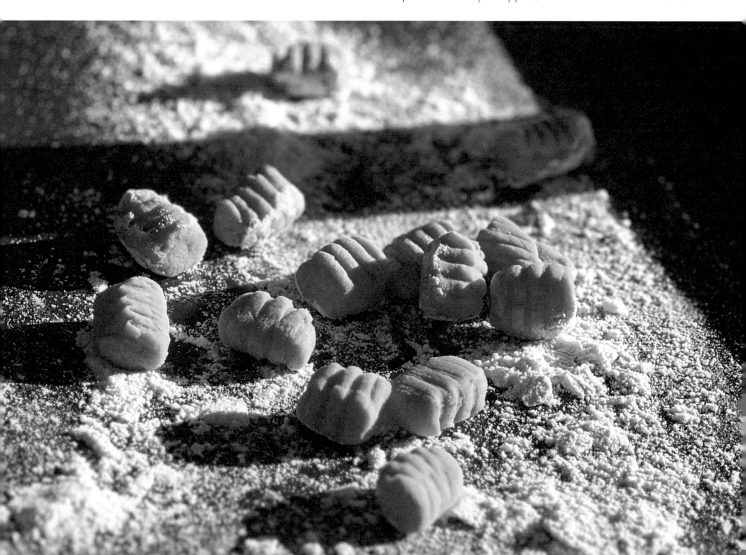

cheese, salt, cracked black pepper, and a pinch of nutmeg until the flavoring is to your liking. Taste it. Then, add 1 egg yolk to the potato, making a more cohesive dough that is easier to work with. It is a good starting point if you are just learning the technique.

> *Fun Fact: Hens that are given feed full of yellow-orange pigments will lay eggs with darker yolks.*

> *Note: There is a potato gnocchi recipe in my cookbook, Food That Will Gather Your Family. This requires Russet potatoes and uses all-purpose flour.*

Step Four: Now sprinkle on the flour in thirds, working the flour into the sweet potatoes with the scraper. Use the entire surface area of the board. Chop it all together until it starts to form into a dough-like texture.

Step Five: At this point, you will see a dough literally forming. Work the dough until it is uniform in color and perfectly combined.

> *Note: You may need 1 additional tablespoon (or more) of flour. The dough should not be tacky, if so, add 1 tablespoon at a time of flour until the dough is no longer sticky.*

Step Six: Form the dough into a loaf about 4 inches wide and 2 inches tall. Chop and roll! Using the pastry scraper, chop off 10 large chunks from the loaf. Add excess flour to the board. Then roll each piece with your hands into a dowel, about 14 inches long and ¾-inch wide.

> *Note: If you are using regular flour and not gluten-free flour, then you must cover the loaf and rest it for at least 20 minutes. This is an important step.*

Step Seven: Cut the dowel into 1-inch bite-sized pieces using the pastry scrapper. They should look like tiny pillows. You can stop here and boil them. If you choose to decorate them, move onto **Step Eight**.

Step Eight: You can use a gnocchi board to roll the gnocchi and make the lined indentations, or you can use a fork and roll each gnocchi to make indentations. Gnocchi can be shaped many ways.

Step Nine: Add about 1 tablespoon of table salt (or more) to boiling water. This is an important step as the salt will flavor the gnocchi (or pasta). The water can be on a medium to low boil, not a rolling boil. Toss in 1 or 2 gnocchi to test the cooking time. The gnocchi will float to the top when they are done. I typically cook them for about 2 minutes, then fish them out with a spider strainer.

Taste the gnocchi after 2 minutes. They should be done. Once you have figured out your cooking time, pile the gnocchi onto the spider strainer and put them into the boiling water. Give the water a quick stir so they do not stick together. Add the lid to be sure the water boils, then you can take it off. When they rise to the top, take them out with the strainer (do not dump into a colander; they will break) and transfer them right onto the plate with prepared sauce. When you bite into a fluffy, airy pillow of goodness, you are transported to Italy in one delicious bite.

Some pairing ideas are asparagus and basil in the spring with a light cream sauce. Asparagus starts to show up in mid to late April on the East Coast. On the West Coast, particularly in parts of California, asparagus pops out of the ground about a month earlier.

For a heartier bite in the winter months, try fresh sage leaves with creminis or button mushrooms cooked in butter or browned butter. Add a little cream or crème fraiche off the heat. The best way to attain crispy mushrooms is to sauté them in a hot skillet with a little oil. There is nothing better than crispy, slightly salty mushrooms.

> *Fun fact: Cremini mushrooms are sometimes referred to as mini bella, baby bellas, or portobellini mushrooms.*

POTATO DUMPLINGS

INGREDIENTS:

- 4 large Russet potatoes, scrubbed and rinsed
- 1 cup all-purpose flour (or gluten-free flour)
- 1 teaspoon onion powder
- ½ teaspoon table salt
- Cracked black pepper to taste
- 1 tablespoon dried parsley flakes
- 1 large egg, premixed
- 1 tablespoon extra virgin olive oil
- ¼ cup warm water
- 2–3 tablespoons salted butter (or more)
- Sea salt as needed to flavor
- Potato ricer (or potato masher)
- Wood pastry board
- Large pot
- Medium-sized non-stick frying pan

Step One: Scrub the potatoes and thoroughly rinse and dry them. Potatoes hold a fair amount of dirt on the skin. It's best to choose organic to avoid unnecessary pesticides. Choose what you have available at your local market.

Step Two: Pierce the potatoes with the prongs of a fork, about 3–4 times. Place them in the microwave to cook or in the oven at 425 degrees for about 1 hour or longer. Do not wrap in foil. Once potatoes are fork tender, they are ready to work with. Allow them to cool.

Step Three: Peel the potatoes. Rough chop them and add big chunks to the potato ricer. If you do not have a potato ricer, mash potatoes on the wood board using a fork or in a bowl using a potato masher. Discard any skin.

Step Four: Once the potatoes are thoroughly mashed into fine bits, add them to a large bowl along with flour, seasonings, a premixed egg, olive oil, and warm water. Mix until the dough forms together. When you squeeze the dough, it should stick together.

Note: Whichever gluten-free flour you are using, be sure it contains xanthan gum, so it holds everything together. I have tested this recipe using regular flour and King Arthurs' Baking Company's Gluten-Free Measure For Measure Flour and they are both very good.

Step Five: Form the dough into a large loaf about 9 inches long by 5–6 inches wide, cover with a clean dish towel. Rest dough 20 minutes. In the meantime, fill the pot with water and bring it to a boil.

Step Six: Cut the loaf into 8 (1-inch) slices. Cut each slice into thirds and make 30 balls of dough. Press each ball down to form a dumpling.

Step Seven: Once the water comes to a boil, add ⅓ of the dumplings at a time (about 10). Cooking them in batches will ensure they cook through. The dumplings are done once they float to the top and then cook an additional minute. Total cooking time is about 3–4 minutes. Be sure to reduce heat so it's not on a rapid boil.

Step Eight: Add ½ tablespoon of butter to the pan and heat on low. Strain out the dumplings with a spider strainer or slotted spoon. Place onto a plate. Add 6 dumplings into the frying pan at a time. Heat 1 minute a side and flip and heat an additional 1 minute a side. Cook until golden brown. If they feel mushy, continue to cook longer and raise heat. Add more butter to the pan and continue to cook dumplings.

Step Nine: Add sea salt to the dumplings, serve, and enjoy! Dip in sour cream with chopped chives or eat them warm from the pan.

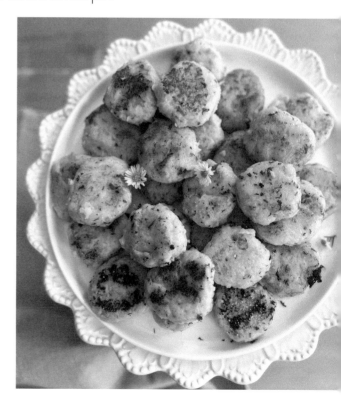

MUSHROOM RAGU
WITH PAPPARDELLE

SERVES 6

A traditional Italian ragu is a meat-based sauce made with vegetables and served with a pappardelle, tagliatelle, or fettucine pasta. Mine is a vegetable-based option and is on the lighter side made with a combination of mushrooms, carrots, celery, onion, and lots of seasonings in a rich tomato sauce. This has layers of delicious flavors with the addition of butter, red wine, stock, and fresh herbs. Pancetta is optional if you are not living a vegetarian lifestyle.

INGREDIENTS:

- 3–4 carrots, peeled and rough chopped
- 3–4 celery stalks, peeled and rough chopped
- ½ large yellow onion, diced
- 3–4 garlic cloves
- 2 tablespoons salted butter
- 4 tablespoons chopped pancetta (optional)
- 1 (24-ounce) package plus 1 (8-ounce) package baby bella mushrooms, about 10 cups chopped
- ½ cup beef stock (or vegetable stock)
- ¼ cup cabernet sauvignon (or any red wine)
- 2 cups crushed tomato sauce
- 3–4 bay leaves

- 1 cup whole (or low-fat milk), warmed
- Ground sea salt
- A good quality extra virgin olive oil
- 4 tablespoons tomato paste (optional)
- Red chili flakes (optional)
- 16 ounces pappardelle, tagliatelle, or fettuccine (or gluten-free pasta)
- Garnish: chopped fresh parsley (or basil ribbons), and Parmigiano-Reggiano cheese
- High-speed blender
- Medium-sized non-stick frying pan for carrots, celery, onion, and garlic
- Large enameled coated cast-iron skillet for mushrooms and ragu sauce

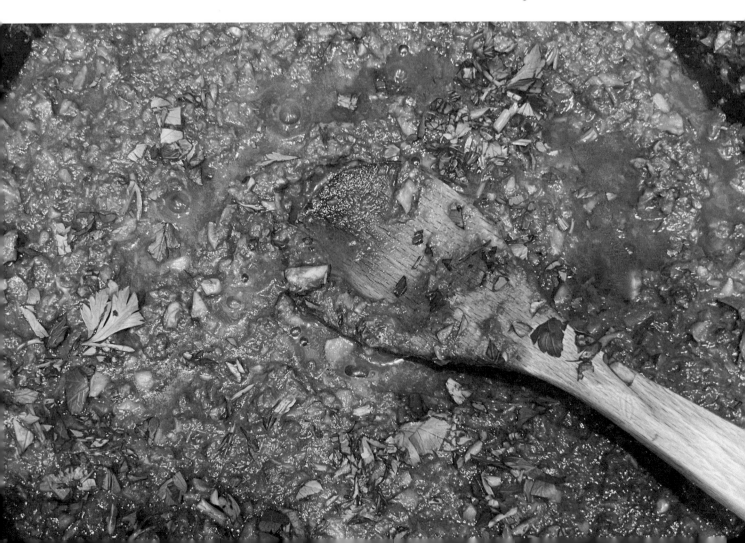

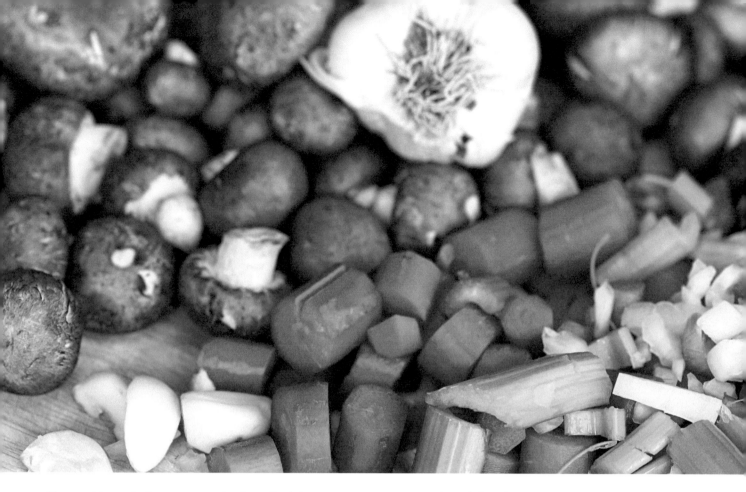

Thoroughly wash the carrots and celery. Peel the carrots and celery and rough chop them. Set them aside. Thoroughly rinse the mushrooms in a colander and place them onto a clean dish towel. Clean and wipe every mushroom to get rid of any dirt. Allow them to air-dry.

Make the Mushroom Ragu.

In the high-blender, add the rough-chopped carrots, celery, diced onions, and garlic cloves. Mince, about 2 minutes. Use the agitator stick.

Note: The minced carrots, celery, onion, and garlic should measure roughly 4 cups.

Add the butter and a drizzle of olive oil to the medium-sized non-stick frying pan. Transfer the vegetables to the pan and sauté for about 8 minutes on medium heat until they just start to brown. Be sure to season with a little salt.

Note: If you are adding the pancetta, add it to the pan with the butter, allow it to cook for 6 minutes until browned, and then transfer the carrot-celery mixture to the pan.

In the meantime, using a good chef's knife, finely chop all the mushrooms including stems. Add a good drizzle of olive oil to the large skillet and add the mushrooms along with a sprinkle of sea salt. Allow the mushrooms to

simmer and cook for about 20 minutes or longer. Cook the mushrooms in batches to not overcrowd the pan.

Note: Feel free to use a combination of mushrooms like shitake and baby bella mushrooms.

Once the mushrooms are done, add the vegetables into the pan with the mushrooms along with the stock. Off the heat, add the stock, wine, tomato sauce, bay leaves, and warmed milk. Red chili flakes are optional.

Note: To avoid the milk from curdling, keep heat on low.

Let this simmer for 30 minutes or longer on low heat. The liquid will reduce as you cook it. If you find it's still runny, you may add the tomato paste.

Prepare the pasta according to package directions. Reserve some pasta water. Combine the cooked pasta with the ragu sauce. Serve with chopped parsley, or basil ribbons, and a shaving of Parmigiano-Reggiano cheese.

Nutrition tip: Mushrooms like shitakes are powerhouse foods and good for brain health. They are very low in calories. One cup of raw chopped mushrooms equals 16 calories. It is highly recommended to eat mushrooms cooked versus raw. Learn more about improving brain health in the Q & A section with Samara at the end of this book.

RED LENTIL BOLOGNESE
WITH CREAMY PARMESAN POLENTA
(Gluten Free)

SERVES 4–6

INGREDIENTS:

- 1 cup dry red (or brown) lentils
- 4–5 fresh garlic cloves, finely diced
- Red chili flakes to taste
- 2 carrots, peeled and chopped
- 2 celery stalks, peeled and chopped
- 1 medium sweet onion, chopped
- 1 (4.6-ounce) tube tomato paste
- ¾ cup red wine
- 1 (28-ounce) can San Marzano whole peeled tomatoes
- 1 package baby bella mushrooms (or shitake mushrooms), about 2 ¼ cups sliced
- Sea salt and cracked black pepper to taste
- A good quality extra virgin olive oil
- Garnish: basil ribbons (or fresh parsley)
- Balsamic glaze, about 1 teaspoon (optional)
- High-speed blender
- Enamel-coated cast-iron skillet to cook mushrooms
- Medium-sized non-stick frying pan
- Strainer

Creamy Parmesan Polenta:

- 3 tablespoons salted butter
- 1 shallot, diced
- 3 fresh garlic cloves, finely chopped
- ½ cup whole milk, warmed
- 3 ½ cups chicken stock (or vegetable stock)
- 1 cup stone-ground cornmeal
- ½ cup creamed corn, canned (gluten free)
- ½ cup grated Parmigiano-Reggiano (or parmesan cheese)
- A good quality extra virgin olive oil
- Ground sea salt and cracked black pepper to taste
- Medium-sized non-stick pan
- Enamel-coated cast-iron skillet

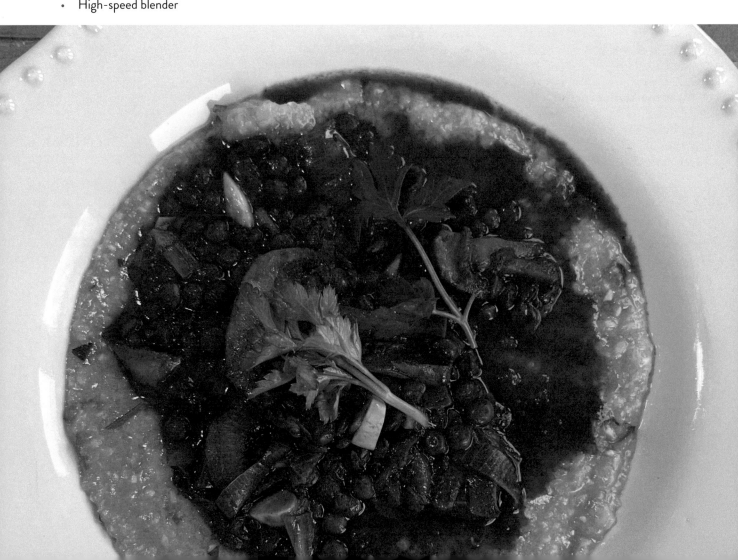

Start by precooking the lentils. You will need about 2 ½ cups of cooked red lentils. If you cannot find red lentils, you may use brown lentils which will just give this dish an earthy undertone.

Next, add a few drizzles of olive oil in the non-stick frying pan. Add the diced garlic. Heat on medium-low until translucent, about 5 minutes. Add a few shakes of red chili flakes to toast them.

In the meantime, mince the chopped carrots, celery, and onions in the blender. You do not want any chunks to remain. This is a great tip I learned from an Italian chef to add the chopped vegetables to the blender to mince when preparing a Bolognese sauce.

Add the mixture to the non-stick pan with the garlic and continue to heat on medium for about 8 minutes. The combination of carrots, celery, onions, and garlic creates the flavor base for this delicious sauce and is known in Italy as the sofrito.

> *Sofrito is an aromatic flavor base composed of sautéed carrots, celery, and onion that forms the foundation of many soups, stews, sauces, and braises throughout Italian cuisine.*

Add the tube of tomato paste to the mixture. Heat for an additional 8 minutes on medium heat. Remove from the heat, then deglaze the pan with red wine. The mixture will become a deep red color. Return the pan to the heat and cook for 8 more minutes on low heat.

Note: Wine is flammable, so use extra caution. Another reason why you should have a fire extinguisher in the kitchen.

Rinse the blender. Strain the whole peeled tomatoes through a strainer to reserve the liquid. You can use the back of a wooden spoon to press the liquid out. Dump the tomatoes into a colander to rinse out seeds. Place the whole peeled tomatoes in the blender and blend for 1 minute. Add the tomatoes to the sofrito mixture and heat for 8 minutes. Season with salt and black pepper.

Note: I prefer to rinse out the tomato seeds because they are a little bitter, but you can skip this step. Reserve the liquid either way.

Strain the lentils, add them to the mixture in the pan, and simmer for 20–25 minutes.

In the meantime, add a drizzle of oil to the skillet. Add the sliced mushrooms and a sprinkle of sea salt. Heat on medium-high heat until the mushrooms are browned, then add these to the pan with the lentil-vegetable mixture.

Once all the ingredients are combined, taste it and decide if you need more seasonings. Add the balsamic glaze.

While the flavors meld, prepare the creamy polenta.

Make the Creamy Parmesan Polenta.

Add the butter to the skillet. Dice the shallots and finely chop the garlic. Add them to the pan with the butter and heat on low for 5–7 minutes. Add a sprinkle of sea salt.

Next, heat ½ cup milk in a microwave-safe bowl in microwave for 30 seconds. Add warmed milk to the pan with 3 ½ cups of stock. Allow this to come to a gentle boil, then immediately whisk in 1 cup of cornmeal and lower heat to medium. Whisk continuously to fully incorporate the cornmeal and get out any lumps, about 3–5 minutes. Add the creamed corn (to make this extra creamy), and heat for 15 minutes on medium-low heat. Season with more ground sea salt and cracked black pepper to taste.

Note: There are brands that make gluten-free creamed corn. If you cannot find it, just omit it.

After 15 minutes, add the parmesan cheese. Heat on low for 5 more minutes. If it continues to thicken and you want to loosen it, add a splash of milk. Top with more cracked black pepper.

To serve, pour 1 ladle-sized spoonful of polenta into a medium-sized bowl and add in a heaping ladle of Red Lentil Bolognese Sauce. Garnish with chopped fresh parsley or basil chiffonade.

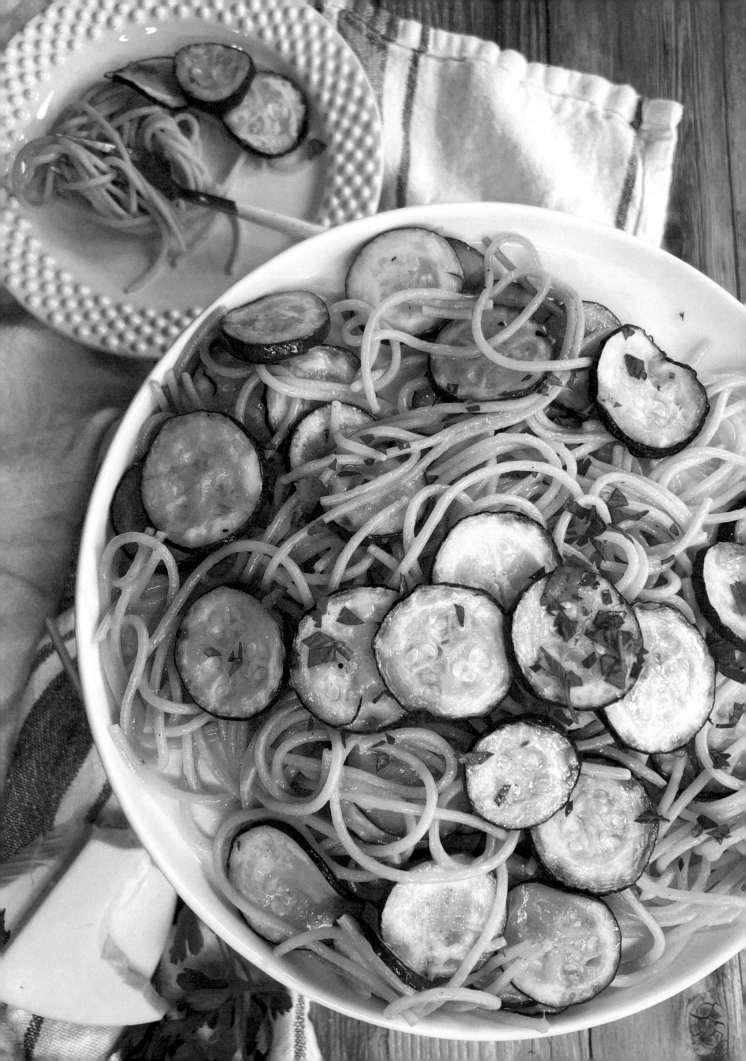

PASTA NERANO
"SPAGHETTI ALLA NERANO"
by Chef Rosangela

I am very blessed to have such amazing professionally-trained chefs for friends. Chef Rosangela graciously offered this recipe for me to feature in this cookbook. We both share Italian heritage, love to cook, and eat! Rosangela has a finesse for creating delicious recipes that she showcases at her bistro, Capri Italian Bakery and Bistro, Maple Ridge, British Columbia, Canada.

Pasta Nerano, also known as Spaghetti alla Nerano, is an Italian pasta dish invented in the Italian village of Nerano, Italy, on the Sorrento peninsula. Anyone who travels to Italy and vacations along the Amalfi Coast knows that you must eat this when you go. Now, if you cannot get to Italy anytime soon, you will have this recipe to enjoy, and know that someday you'll order it and enjoy it overlooking the cliffs along the Amalfi Coast sipping an aperitif while you wait.

Rosangela spent many summers in Nerano, Italy. To get to the beach, or any place in this vertical city, you must take a seemingly never-ending flight of stairs. We both agree, the Amalfi Coast is truly the most enchanting place to visit. This is a 3-ingredient meal, brought together with the starchy pasta water to create a light, creamy, and delicious dish reminiscent of the quaint and picturesque town of Nerano, Italy. Mangia!

INGREDIENTS:

- 2 lbs. zucchini, thinly sliced widthwise (about 3 medium zucchinis)
- ½ lb. shredded Provolone Del Monaco (or half aged Pecorino Romano and half Caciocavallo)
- ½ cup extra virgin olive oil
- 1 lb. spaghetti (or gluten-free spaghetti)
- Basil chiffonade or basil ribbons (or chopped fresh parsley)
- 1 fresh garlic clove
- Ground sea salt
- Medium-sized non-stick pan
- Tongs

Add half the olive oil to the pan and swirl it around to completely cover the bottom. Allow this to heat for 5 minutes on medium. Fry the zucchini slices in the olive oil until golden brown, add sea salt, then flip to the other side and cook until golden. Drain on a paper towel. Do this in batches.

Add the remaining olive oil to the pan. Smash a garlic clove and add it to the olive oil. Heat on medium until golden and discard. This will infuse some flavor into the oil.

Cook the pasta according to package directions until it is a few minutes away from al dente. Reserve 1 cup of pasta water.

Place the pan on the back burner to avoid splashing hot oil and add the pasta to the oil and stir continually. Then add the pasta water, most of the zucchini (reserve some for plating) and a few basil leaves.

Through the process of continually mixing the water and oil, two immiscible liquids, the pasta will become luxuriously creamy. Once the pasta starts becoming creamy, turn the heat off and slowly start adding the cheese, stirring between every addition. Make sure the cheese emulsifies with the starchy pasta water and becomes creamy by continually stirring.

Note: If you cannot find Provolone Del Monaco, use a combination of aged Pecorino Romano and Caciocavallo cheeses.

Once all the cheese is fully incorporated, you are ready to plate. Garnish with the remaining zucchini slices and basil leaves. Buon Appetito!

Gardening tip: Plant zucchini and be sure to give it a fair amount of room to grow. It can easily take over the entire garden. Best to handle with gloves as the vines are very prickly.

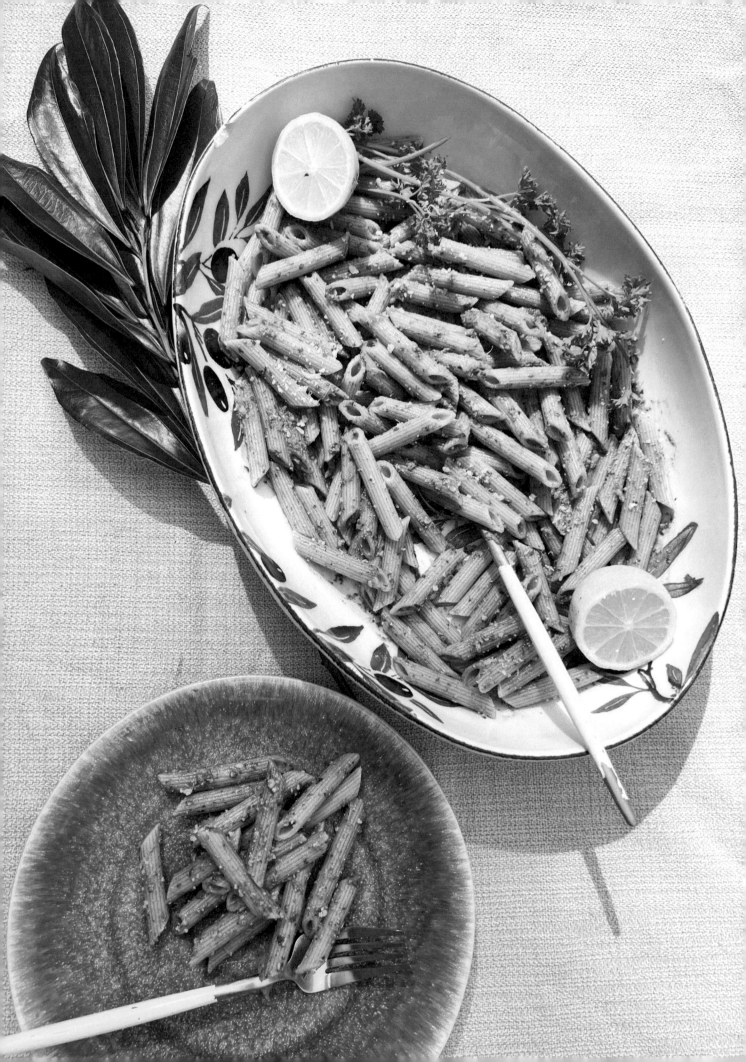

PESTO PENNE PASTA

SERVES 4

Jack and I worked together to develop this recipe. He and I love making pesto with fresh basil from our garden. We use what's on hand to avoid food waste and will pull in some spinach or arugula depending on what's in the fridge.

Eating seasonally, meaning eating what's fresh and in season and at peak flavor is something we do especially in the summer, when we turn to our garden for inspiration. We pick the basil from our garden and use it to make pesto. It is farm-to-table cooking at its best.

You can use any greens you have on hand to make pesto: kale, arugula, basil, parsley, or a combination of them. Nuts like pine nuts, walnuts, or even seeds can also be added. In addition, to make it creamier and to add a little more protein, add some chick peas and blend into the pesto mixture.

INGREDIENTS:

- 4 cups fresh baby spinach, packed (or kale)
- 1 cup fresh basil leaves (or more)
- ¼ cup finely grated Parmigiano-Reggiano (or parmesan cheese)
- ¼ cup extra virgin olive oil
- 1 teaspoon minced garlic (or 1 whole garlic clove)
- 1 lemon, squeezed (or 2 tablespoons lemon juice)
- ½ (1 lb.) bag penne rigate pasta (or linguine, or gluten-free pasta)
- Salt to taste
- ¼ cup reserved pasta water
- Medium-sized pot
- High-speed blender (or food processor)

Add the spinach and basil to the blender, along with the parmesan, olive oil, garlic, and lemon juice. Blend for about 1 minute, using the agitator stick. It should be little chunky, but all the spinach leaves should be broken into tiny bits. Taste the pesto and add salt to your liking. Pour the pesto into a medium-sized bowl.

Once the water comes to a boil, salt it to infuse some flavor into the pasta. Add the pasta and make it according to box or package directions. Reserve ¼ cup of water or more.

Strain the pasta and add it to the bowl with the pesto. Do not rinse pasta. Mix well to fully coat the pasta. Add a little shaving more of cheese. As the pasta sits it will start to dry out a little; use a little drizzle of the reserved pasta water to loosen.

Note: Adding the pesto to a hot pan will darken the hue. You want it to be bright and fresh, so always do it off the heat.

Serve with bread and enjoy!

If you want to double the recipe and make more pesto, add leftover pesto to a jar, and cover in the fridge for up to 3 days. Add a little olive oil to the top so it doesn't brown.

Chef tip: Twirl pasta using a large pasta fork inside a soup ladle and gently pour onto a plate for a beautiful presentation, and proper portioning of any linguine or spaghetti dish. Learn more about portioning in the Q & A section with Samara at the end of this book.

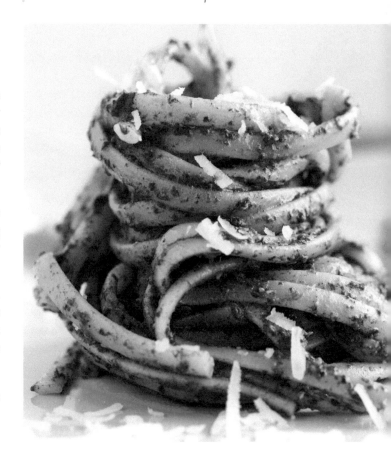

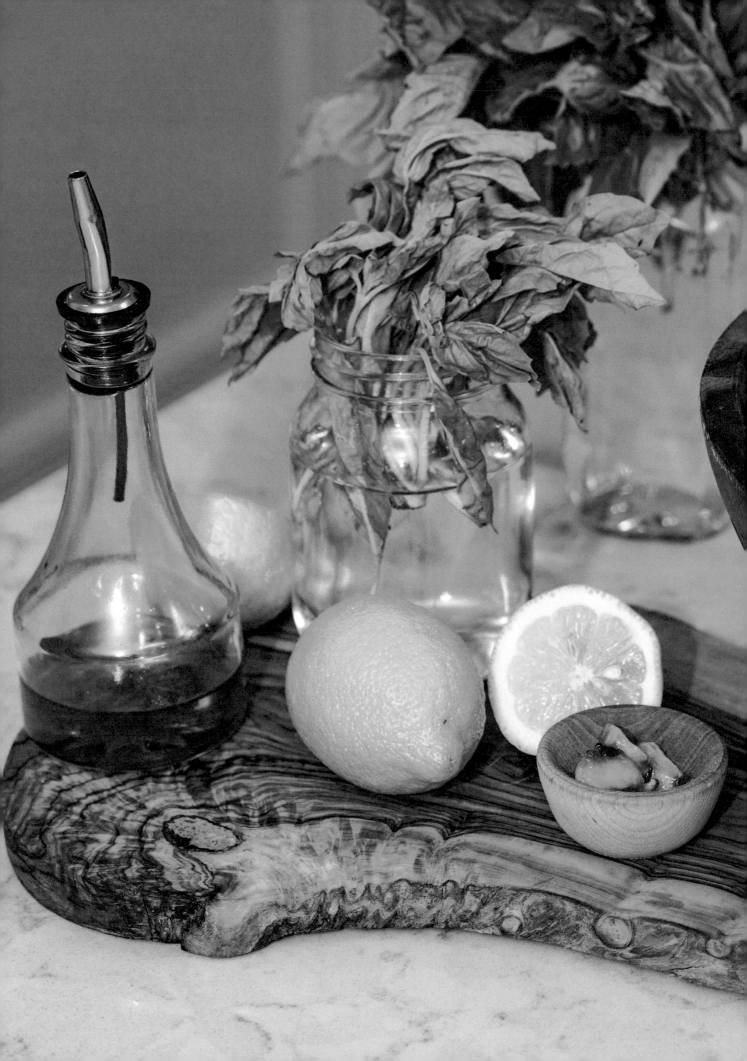

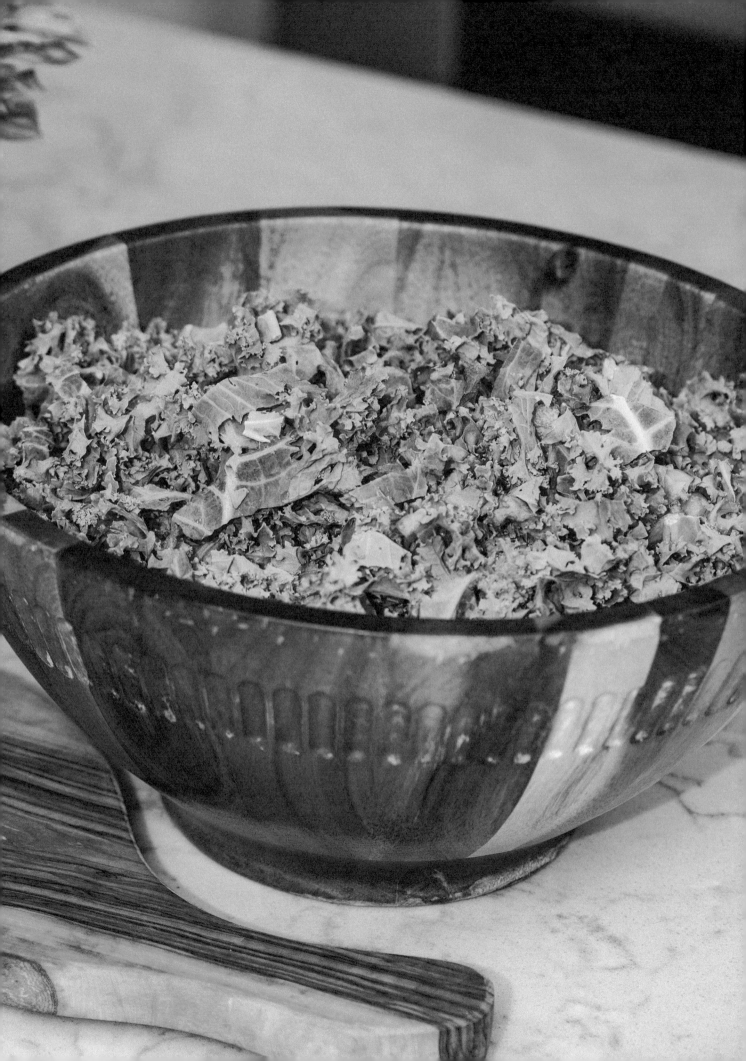

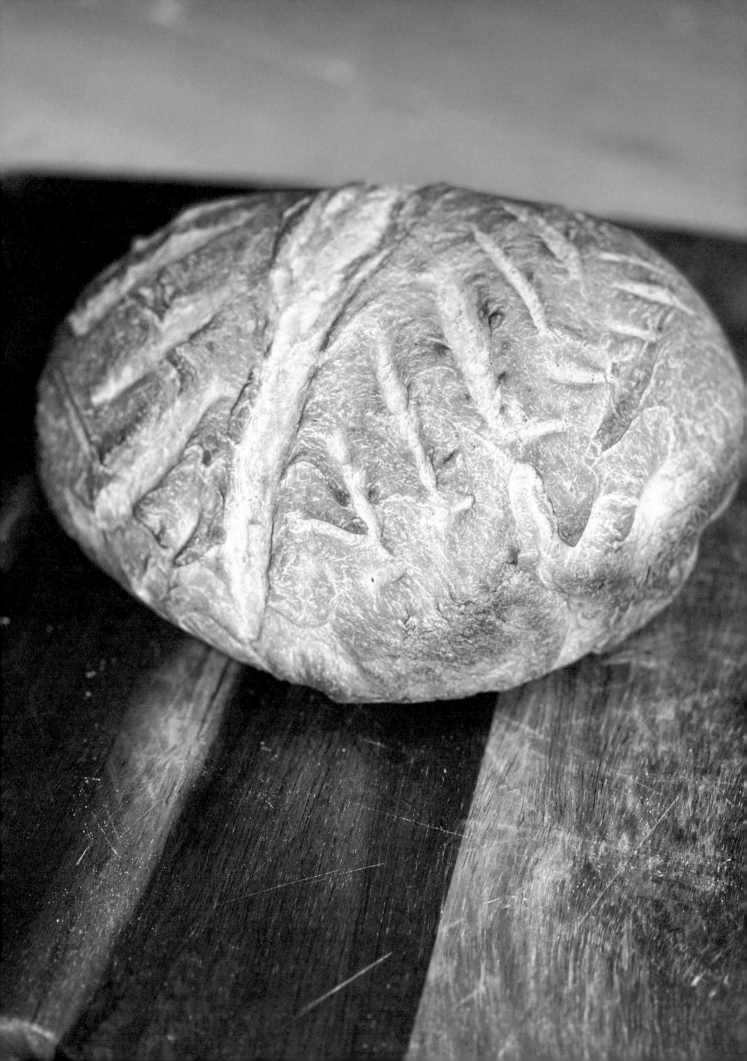

PIZZAS
AND BREADS

BROCCOLI PIZZA CRUST
(Gluten Free)

SICILIAN PAN PIZZA

CAULIFLOWER PIZZA CRUST
WITH PROSCIUTTO, PEPPERONI, AND HOT HONEY
(Gluten Free)

TWISTED BREAD RINGS

OLIVE LOAF BREAD

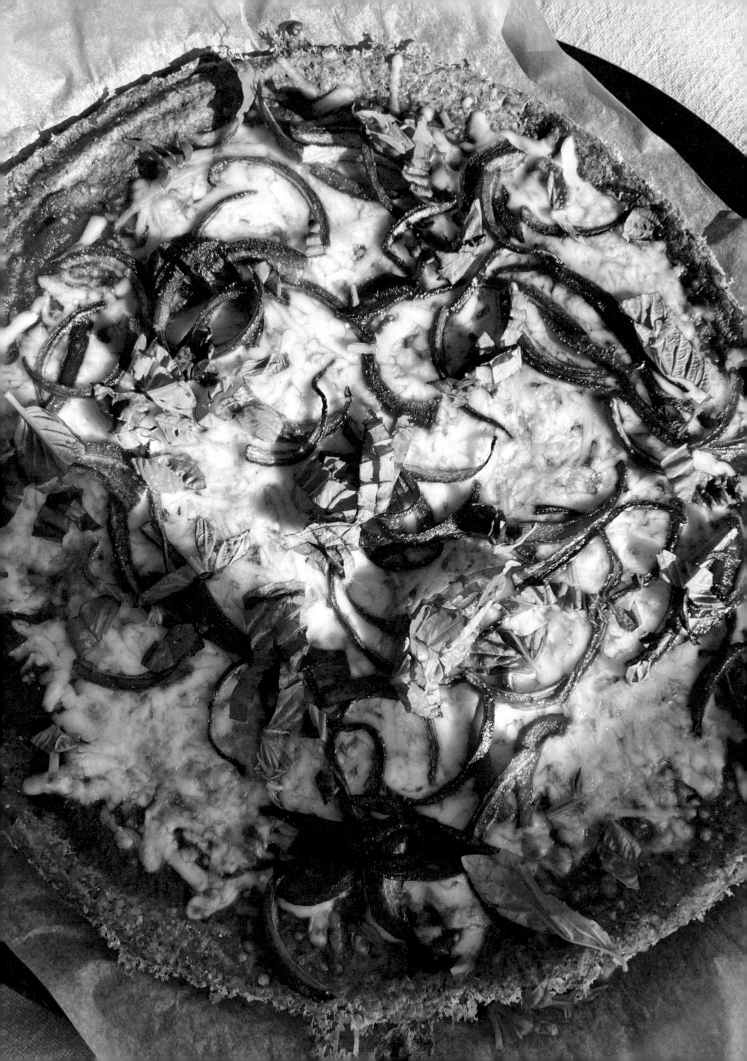

BROCCOLI PIZZA CRUST
(Gluten Free)

1 MEDIUM PIZZA | SERVES 3-4

INGREDIENTS:

- 8 cups broccoli florets, cooked
- ¼ cup finely grated parmesan cheese (or more)
- 1 large egg plus 1 egg white
- ½ cup plus 1 tablespoon King Arthur Baking Company's Gluten Free Pizza Flour (or all-purpose flour)
- Garlic powder and salt to taste
- Cheesecloth
- High-speed blender
- 2 medium-sized round pizza pans (1 for baking, 1 for flipping)

Pizza Toppings:

- ½ cup jarred tomato sauce
- 1 cup part-skim shredded mozzarella cheese
- A sprinkling of Pecorino Romano cheese
- ½ red onion, thinly sliced
- 1 teaspoon balsamic glaze (optional)
- Garlic powder and sea salt to taste

Preheat oven to 425 degrees.

Boil the broccoli until fork tender. Once cooled, add it to a blender and mash completely with the agitator stick. Spoon the mashed broccoli into the cheesecloth (over the sink), and gently squeeze to strain out any excess liquid. This step is highly recommended, especially if you boil the broccoli as it will retain a lot of moisture.

Next, add the mixture back into the blender with the parmesan cheese and eggs. Mix until combined. Or you can mix it by hand. Dump the mixture into a medium-sized bowl. Add the flour, garlic powder, and salt. Mix with a spoon until a cohesive dough has formed. If it's tacky, add 1 teaspoon of flour at a time.

Note: You may also substitute the flour for ground flaxseed (or flax meal).

Spread the broccoli crust onto the parchment-lined round pizza pan. Add a second piece of parchment paper to the top and smooth it out, evenly spreading the broccoli dough, about ¾-inch thickness. Gently peel back the top piece of parchment paper.

Bake the crust for 18 minutes or longer. Then top the crust with a new piece of parchment paper, place the other pizza pan on top. With oven mitts, flip the pizza onto the new pan, carefully peeling back the parchment paper (formerly the bottom of pizza crust), as it will stick a little. Holding the ends of the parchment paper, transfer back to the hot pan.

Bake for 6 minutes or until firm and golden. Then top with tomato sauce, shredded mozzarella cheese, Pecorino Romano cheese, and seasonings. Alternatively, use any toppings of your choice. Bake just until cheese melts, about 6–8 minutes.

Make the Red Onions.

Cut half of a red onion into thin slices and sauté in a non-stick pan with balsamic glaze. Cook about 10 minutes. Top when you finish adding the cheese.

Wait 10 minutes to eat it. You'll find the crust will hold together nicely, and you should be able to hold it like a regular slice of pizza. If the crust is a bit too mushy, reheat until firm. Then immediately transfer to a wood board. The parchment paper will be somewhat wet, and you don't want it to make the pizza soggy.

Nutrition tip: Broccoli, cauliflower, cabbage, kale, bok choy, arugula, chard, and brussel sprouts are cruciferous vegetables. They are easy to find in local markets and are nutrient-rich vegetables providing antioxidant properties.

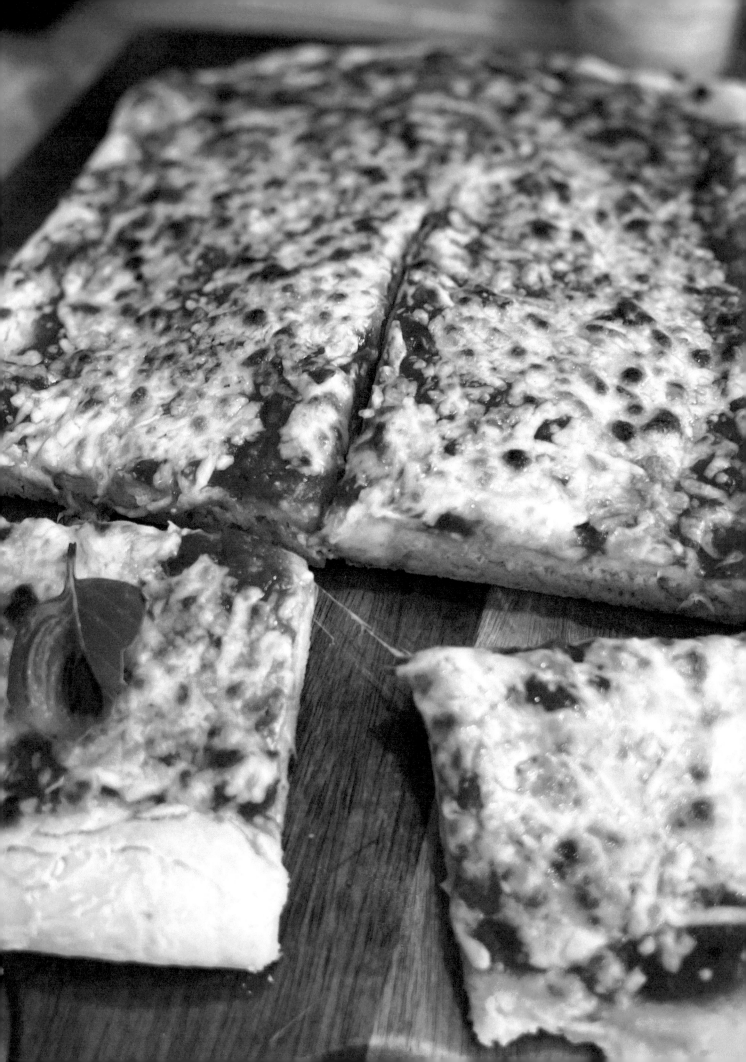

SICILIAN PAN PIZZA
NO KNEAD AND NO YEAST

INGREDIENTS:

- 3 ½ cups all-purpose flour
- 1 tablespoon baking powder
- ½ tablespoon granulated sugar
- 2 ½ teaspoons table salt
- Warm water until dough comes together (about 1 ½ cups)
- 1 ½ tablespoons extra virgin olive oil
- Pan size 13 x 9 inches (1-inch high)
- Non-cooking spray

Pizza Toppings:

- 1 ½ cups jarred tomato sauce
- 1 ½ cups shredded mozzarella cheese
- Ground sea salt
- A drizzle of olive oil
- Mix by hand, preferred method
- Garnish: fresh basil leaves

If you don't have time to wait for your pizza dough to rise, but you want a delicious pizza, make this! You can pull this together in minutes and it's so delicious.

Preheat oven to 425 degrees.

In a large bowl, add the dry ingredients and stir to combine, then slowly drizzle in the water and oil until the dough comes together.

Note: I have made this pizza substituting out 1 ½ cups of the all-purpose flour for whole wheat flour, and it was equally good. You can also substitute the all-purpose flour for gluten-free flour in this recipe.

Dump the dough into a greased pan. Add some olive oil to your hands and press the dough into the pan. Add tomato sauce, mozzarella cheese, and any seasonings you like.

Bake in the oven for about 18 minutes or longer. Check the bottom to be sure it's golden. The last minute, put the broiler on to get the cheese golden brown. This pizza is perfect!

For those of you who have my first cookbook, *Food That Will Gather Your Family*, you know there is a traditional pizza dough recipe in it. It is a wonderful recipe that I use almost every time I make pizza. The only adaptation I have been making more recently is cranking up the heat to 500 degrees and cooking the pizza for a shorter amount of time. Try it!

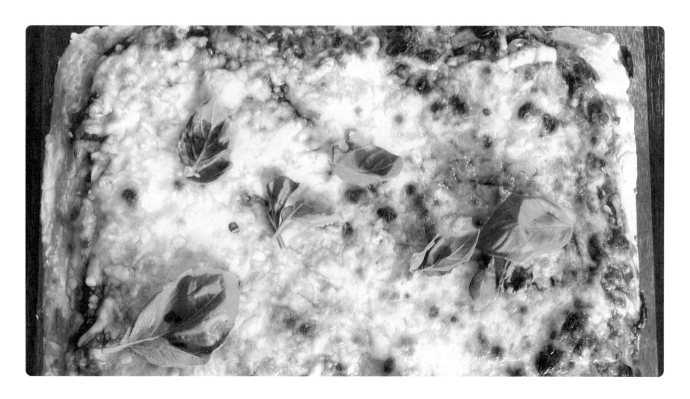

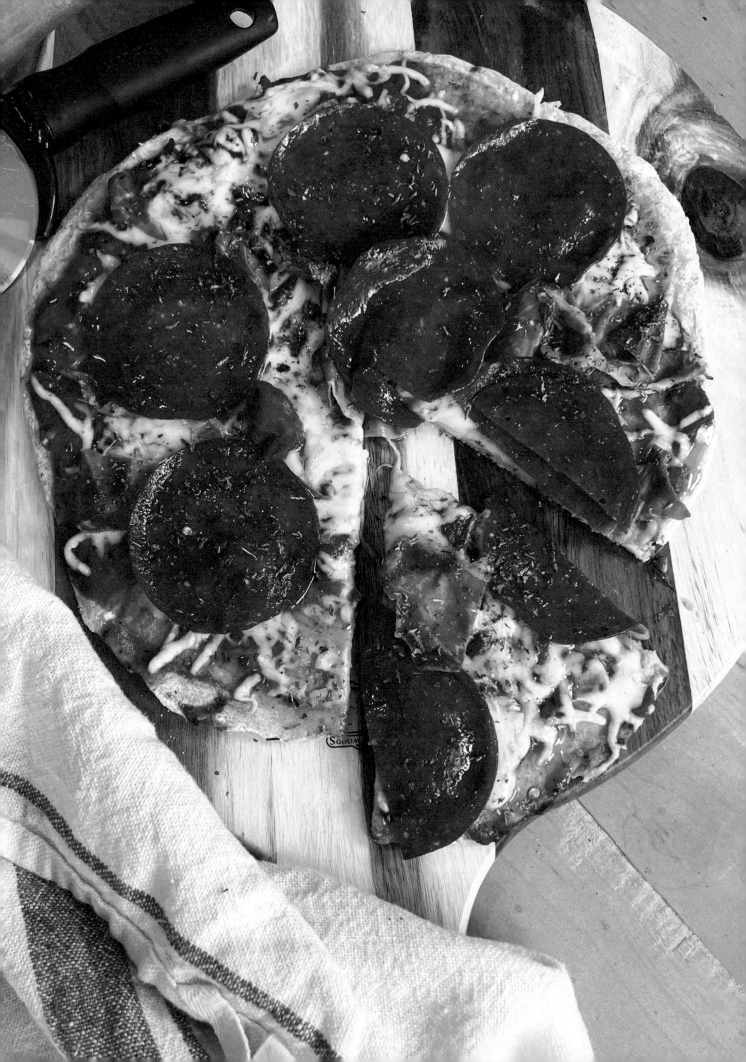

CAULIFLOWER PIZZA CRUST
WITH PROSCIUTTO, PEPPERONI, AND HOT HONEY
(Gluten Free)

INGREDIENTS:

- 1 head steamed cauliflower (yields about 2 ½ cups puréed cauliflower)
- 1 cup plus 3 tablespoons King Arthur Baking Company's Gluten-Free Pizza Flour
- ½ (5.2-ounce) container of garlic and herb soft cheese, room temperature
- Garlic powder to taste
- Italian seasonings to taste
- ¼ teaspoon fine sea salt
- Sprinkle dried parsley flakes
- 1 large egg
- Stand mixer bowl with hook attachment
- Cheesecloth
- High-speed blender
- Excess gluten-free flour for dusting board
- Extra virgin olive oil
- 2 medium-sized round pizza pans (1 for baking, 1 for flipping)
- Wood pastry board

Pizza Toppings:

- ½ cup jarred tomato sauce
- 1 cup shredded part-skim mozzarella cheese
- Italian seasonings and red chili flakes
- 4 slices Prosciutto de Parma
- 5 large slices of pepperoni (may use smaller sized-pepperoni)
- Salt to taste
- Hot honey (or regular honey)

Add the head of cauliflower to a large pot filled with water. Add a tight-fitting lid. Allow it to come to a boil and cook on low heat for about 10 minutes until soft. Next, chop the cauliflower into pieces. Add the cauliflower to the blender. Blend using the agitator stick until smooth.

Next, measure about 2 ½ cups of the puree for this recipe. If you have a little less that is fine. Be sure to thoroughly strain the water from the puréed cauliflower in the cheesecloth to get out any excess liquid. This is a very important step. Add the cauliflower to the stand mixer bowl.

Note: If you use another type of flour blend, be sure it has xanthan gum as an ingredient, otherwise add it to the dough. Alternatively, feel free to make this recipe using all-purpose flour.

In the stand mixer bowl, add the flour (reserve the 3 tablespoons), ½ package of cheese, garlic powder, Italian seasoning, ¼ teaspoon fine sea salt, and parsley flakes to your liking. Last, add the premixed egg and mix on medium until smooth. Add the remaining 3 tablespoons of flour as needed until the dough forms together. If you need 1 more tablespoon of flour, you may add it.

Once the dough forms together, dump it onto a lightly dusted wood board. Knead for a few minutes just to be sure everything is well combined.

Add a drizzle of olive oil to the stand mixer bowl and add the dough back inside. Cover and place in a warm spot for 30 minutes to an hour.

Next, place the dough onto a piece of parchment paper on the wood board. Spread with fingertips, then add a second piece of parchment paper on top and roll out the dough sandwiched between the paper. Slowly take off the top piece and transfer to the pizza round.

Bake in oven at 425 degrees for 8 minutes, then carefully flip onto a new parchment-lined pizza pan using two oven mitts. Bake 4–5 additional minutes until firm.

Then add toppings:

- *Sauce*
- *Mozzarella*
- *Seasonings*
- *Prosciutto and pepperoni*
- *Sprinkle of salt*

Place back directly onto the pizza tin, no parchment paper. I find the parchment paper can make the crust soggy if left too long. Finish baking, about 6 more minutes until the crust is golden. The last minute or 2, drizzle on the hot honey and place on broil. Keep an eye on it.

Not only is this gluten free, but it is a next-level pizza combination.

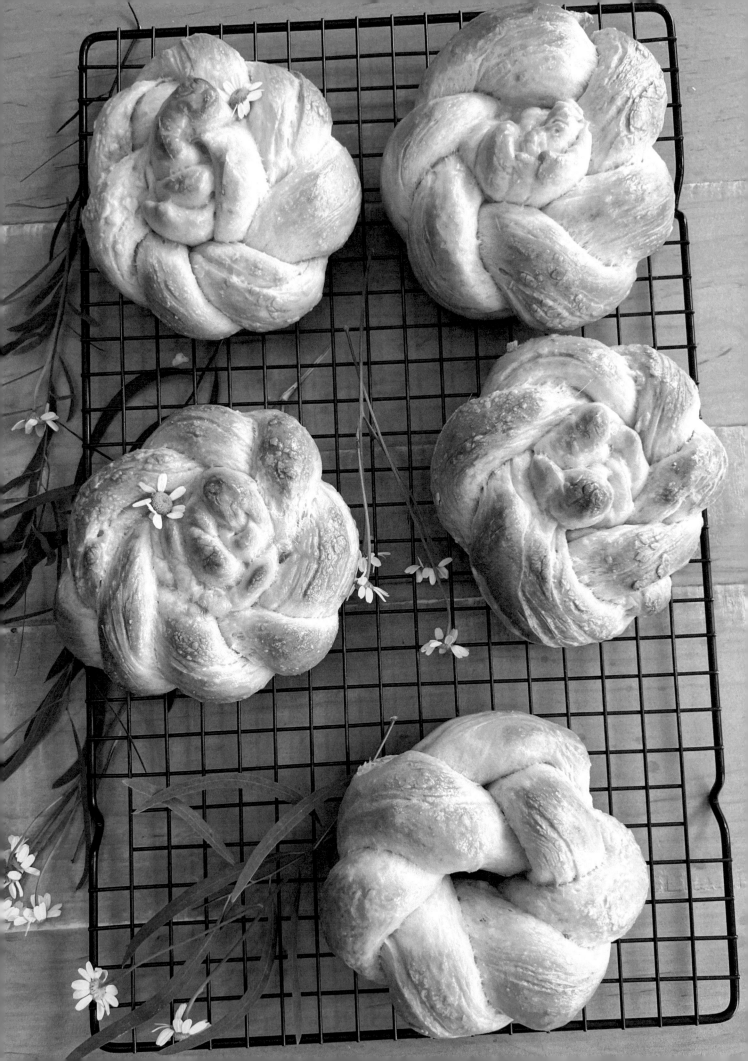

TWISTED BREAD RINGS

MAKES 6 BREAD RINGS

INGREDIENTS:

- 2 ¼ teaspoons rapid-rise yeast dissolved in ¼ cup warm water (or active dry yeast)
- ¼ teaspoon granulated sugar
- 3 cups bread flour
- 1 ½ teaspoons fine sea salt or table salt
- 1 tablespoon extra virgin olive oil
- 1 cup warm water
- 1 egg, premixed
- Wood pastry board
- Rolling pin
- Bench scraper
- Extra flour for dusting
- Pastry brush
- Stand mixer bowl with hook attachment, or mix by hand

Preheat the oven to 350 degrees. This will provide a warm place for our dough to rise. The bread rings will be baked at a higher temperature. I typically do this every time I make bread, bagels, or pizza. After 30 minutes, I turn off the oven.

In a measuring cup, add ¼ cup warm water and stir in the yeast. Mix until foamy. Let it sit for 5 minutes. Add the yeast mixture to the stand mixer bowl with the sugar and mix. Add the flour, salt, olive oil, and remaining water (reserve the egg). Mix until the dough pulls away from the sides of the bowl.

Note: You may use active dry yeast instead of rapid-rise yeast, but the rise time will be longer.

Dump the dough onto a lightly floured wood pastry board, and gently knead the dough for 5 minutes. The stand mixer bowl will have done most of the work. If you are mixing the dough by hand and not using the stand mixer, knead for at least 10 minutes. Add more olive oil to the bottom of the stand mixer bowl, or any metal bowl, and add the dough back. Cover it with a clean dish towel, and place on the stovetop to rise for about 1 hour or longer.

Once the dough has doubled in size, dump it onto a lightly floured wood pastry board.

Preheat the oven to 400 degrees.

Here are the steps to create the most beautiful Twisted Bread with Rose Centers.

Step One: Divide the dough into 12 equal pieces. Take 2 pieces and set them aside to create the roses.

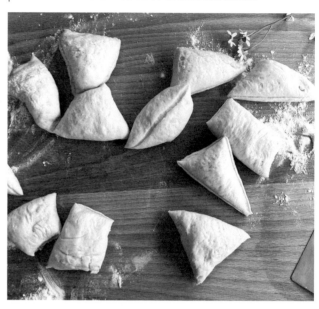

Step Two: Working with 2 pieces at a time, roll each piece into a dowel, about ¾-inch thick and about 10–11 inches long. The size may vary a little. You want them to be even in length.

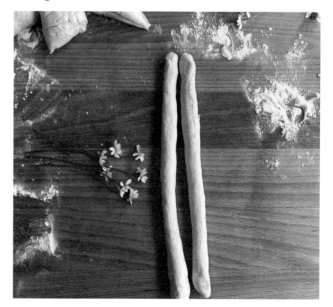

Step Three: Pinch the ends of the 2 dowels together at one end and twist one over the other. Do not seal.

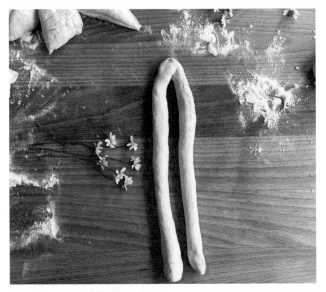

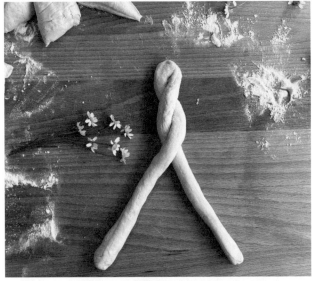

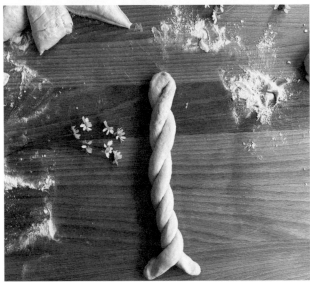

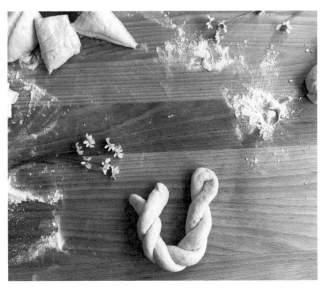

Step Four: Take the end of 1 dowel and thread it through the pinched end (where you started). It's like threading a needle.

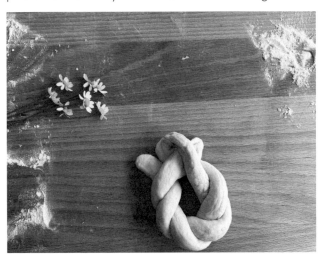

Step Five: Take the other end and pinch it together with the end you threaded. Tuck the newly pinched ends under the ring. Also, tuck the pinched end you started with under. This should form a beautiful, twisted bread ring.

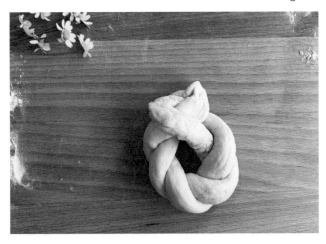

Create the Rose Centers.

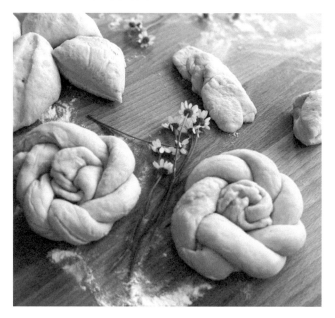

Step Six: Combine the 2 pieces you set aside. Cut 8 equal pieces and roll each into a tiny ball. Working with 4 pieces at a time, roll each piece out flat using the rolling pin. Lay 1 piece on top of the other leaving a little room at the top of each piece. Roll them together vertically.

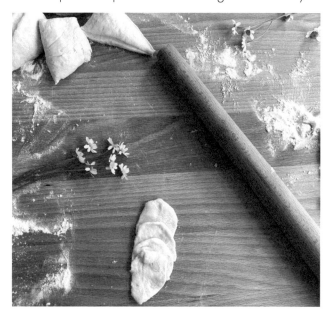

Step Seven: Cut the rolled pieces in half. Now you have 2 roses. Continue this process with the remaining 4 pieces. You will create 4 roses in total to place inside 4 twisted bread rings. 1 will be left without a rose center.

Note: Once you get the hang of making the dough, you can manipulate this recipe and add a little more flour, keeping the yeast the same, but increasing the water to create a cohesive dough. I have tested it with 3 ½ cups of

flour and increased water by ¼ cup more. My rings were slightly larger, and I had enough excess to create 6 rose centers. Practice makes perfect.

Step Eight: Place the rings onto a parchment-lined baking sheet. Cover them with a clean dish towel and allow them to rise, about 10–15 minutes. This is especially important if you added the rose center. You want it to fill in the inside of the bread ring.

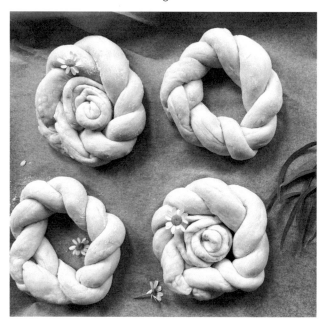

Step Nine: Next, brush each bread ring with the egg wash. Do this twice and be thorough. Bake in the oven on the top rack for 22–24 minutes until golden. Keep an eye on it at around 22 minutes. Oven temperatures can vary.

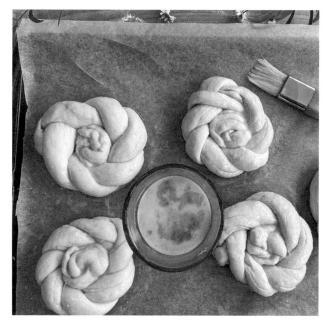

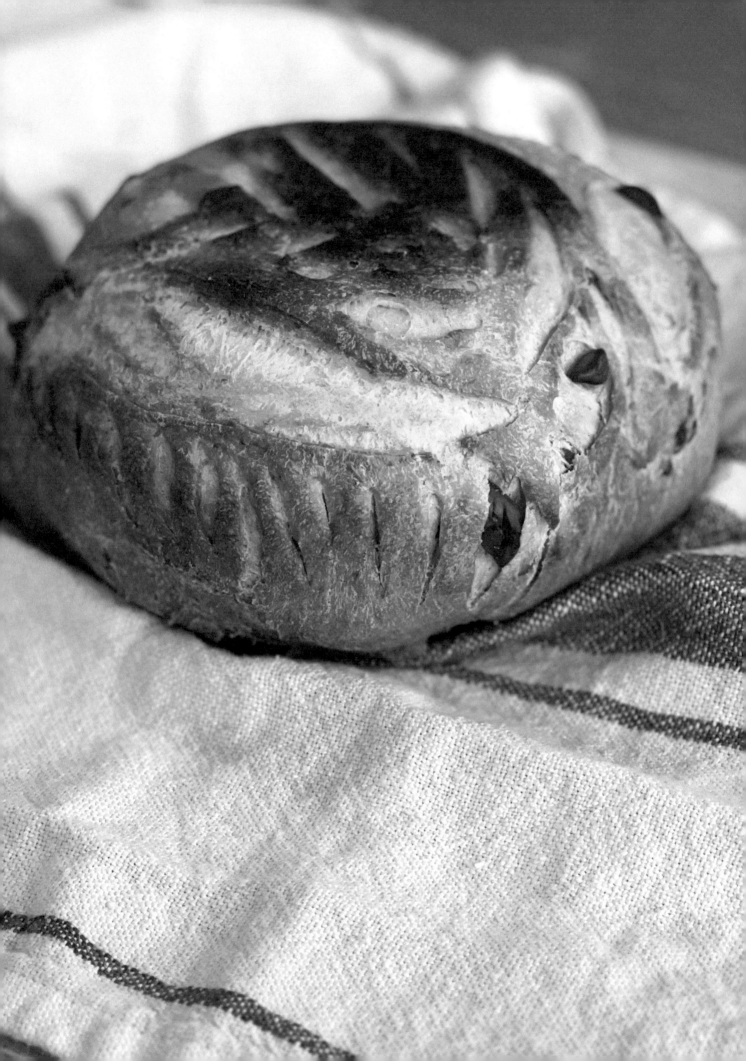

OLIVE LOAF BREAD

INGREDIENTS:

- 2 ¼ teaspoons rapid-rise yeast dissolved in ¼ cup warm water (or active dry yeast)
- 3 cups bread flour, spooned and leveled plus 2–3 tablespoons
- 1 ½ teaspoons sea salt
- 2 tablespoons extra virgin olive oil
- 1 cup warm water, drizzle slowly
- 8–10 colossal green olives stuffed with garlic cloves, finely chopped
- Medium-sized enameled coated cast-iron skillet with tight-fitting lid
- Stand mixer with hook attachment
- Wood pastry board

Preheat the oven to 450 degrees. Heat the skillet in the middle of the oven for about 1 hour *before* baking the bread. This is an important step.

Note: Be sure the cast-iron skillet is large enough. I used 4.5 inches (in height) by 10 inches (in width) enameled coated cast-iron skillet.

Add ¼ cup of water to a measuring cup and stir in yeast until foamy. Pour the mixture into the stand mixer bowl. Allow it to sit for 5–10 minutes, then start making the dough.

Baker's tip: 2 ¼ teaspoons of yeast is equivalent to 1 packet of yeast.

Add 3 cups of bread flour (reserve the 2–3 tablespoons), salt, olive oil, and remaining water into the stand mixer bowl with hook attachment. Mix until the dough starts to come together, then add the diced olives. The dough will be sticky from the olives, so add the remaining 2–3 tablespoons of flour until it is no longer sticky.

Note: I like King Arthur Baking Company's Bread Flour, 12.7% protein for my bread recipes. For a gluten-free alternative, try King Arthur Baking Company's Gluten-Free Measure For Measure Flour. If you are making this bread with another brand of gluten-free flour, be sure it contains xanthan gum otherwise add 1 teaspoon to the bread recipe.

Once the dough pulls away from the sides of the bowl, it is ready. Mix for 5 minutes in the stand mixer bowl until springy, or knead the bread by hand on a lightly floured clean work surface or wood pastry board, about 5–10 minutes.

Baker's tip: Feel free to make this bread and omit the olives.

Dump the dough onto a clean work surface. Lightly oil the stand mixer bowl, then place the dough inside. Cover tightly and place in a warm spot to rise.

Rise time is about 1 hour if you use rapid-rise yeast. If you are using active dry yeast, allow for roughly 1 ½–2 hours of rise time, or until the dough has doubled in size.

After the dough has doubled in size, dump the dough onto a lightly floured work surface or wood pastry board. Stretch, fold, and turn the dough five times. Stretch the dough to the point of resistance. You don't want it to break. Folds should be at the bottom of loaf. Allow dough to rest another 30 minutes, covered.

What is the purpose of folding the dough?

Folding the dough achieves the same function of removing the air bubbles, but it also allows your bread to rise higher once it's baked. These qualities are found in artisan bread.

After 30 minutes, dump the dough onto a lightly floured work surface. Stretch, fold, and turn the dough five more times. Shape dough into a perfectly round loaf so it bakes evenly.

Cut slits to control how the loaf breaks. With practice, this will become artful. Make one long cut down the center and a few artfully placed on either side of the center cut. A good paring knife works well.

Place the dough ball onto the skillet, and heat at 450 degrees for 15 minutes with a tight-fitting lid. Then reduce heat to 375 degrees, bake an additional 23–25 minutes, and check for doneness. It should be golden brown and crispy on the outside and soft and airy on the inside.

It's important to have a tight-fitting lid to encapsulate the steam in the pan, which will then circulate around the bread. The result will be a very crunchy texture on the outside (also known as a crumb).

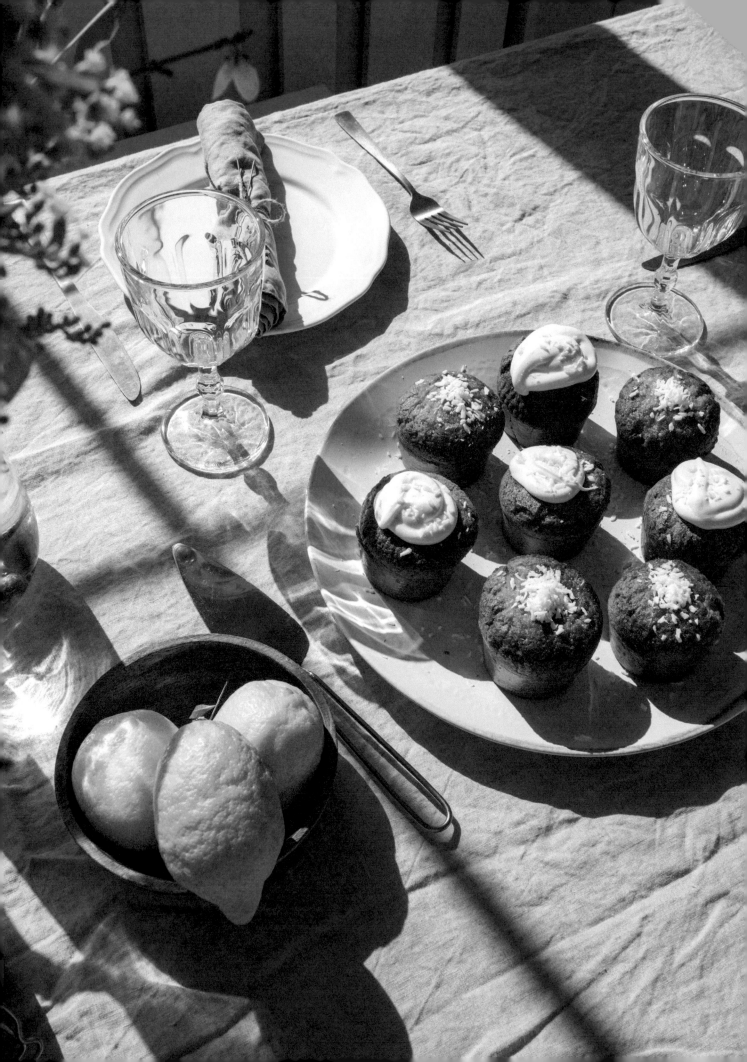

DESSERTS

MINI CHEESECAKES
(Gluten Free)

CHOCOLATE GLAZED OAT-DATE ENERGY BITES
(Gluten Free)

HEALTHY TRUFFLES
(Gluten Free)

CARDAMOM-LAVENDER SNOWBALL COOKIES
(Gluten Free and Nut Free)

HEALTHY MAGIC COOKIE BARS
(Gluten Free)

HEALTHY BROWNIE BITES

CARROT CAKE
(Nut Free)

MINI CHEESECAKES
(Gluten Free)

INGREDIENTS:

Cheesecake Crust:

- 3 cups super-fine almond flour, spooned and leveled
- 1 stick salted butter, melted (8 tablespoons)
- 2 teaspoons vanilla extract
- 2 tablespoons granulated sugar (or light brown sugar)
- Water as needed, about 2 tablespoons

Cheesecake Filling:

- 1 (24-ounce) container cottage cheese, 2%, room temperature
- 1 (8-ounce) container light cream cheese, room temperature
- ½ cup light sour cream, room temperature
- 1 cup powdered sugar (see notes)
- 2 teaspoons clear vanilla extract
- 1 tablespoon lemon, squeezed
- 1 tablespoon cornstarch

- Silicone muffin pan or muffin tin for 12 muffins
- High-speed blender
- Non-stick cooking spray

Blueberry-Blackberry Sauce:

- ¼ cup organic blackberries
- ½ cup mini wild blueberries
- A drizzle of water, about ⅛ cup
- Small non-stick frying pan
- 1 tablespoon sugar (optional)

Raspberry Sauce:

- 1 container fresh organic raspberries (save some for garnish)
- 1 heaping tablespoon raspberry jam
- A drizzle of water, about ⅛ cup
- Small non-stick frying pan
- Strainer
- 1 tablespoon sugar (optional)

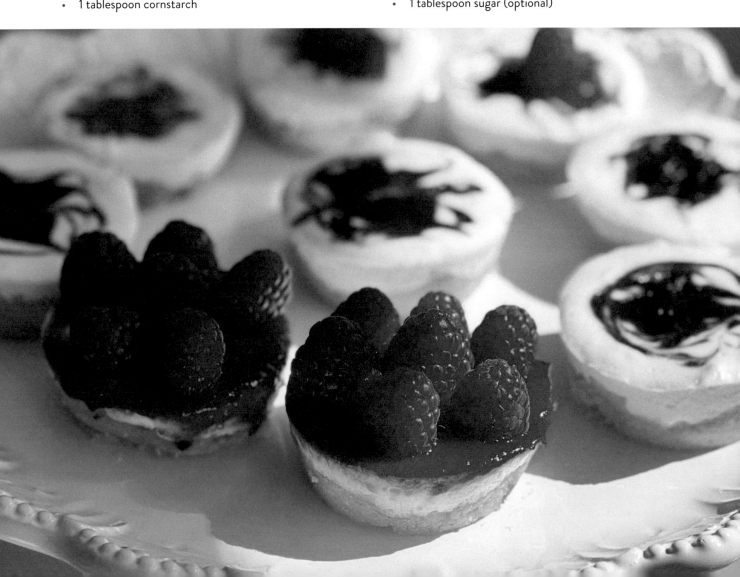

Preheat the oven to 350 degrees. You will be baking the cheesecake on the middle rack. This will ensure it does not brown and bakes evenly. The crust is baked at 350 degrees, but the cheesecake will be baking at 325 degrees. Adjust rack accordingly.

In a bowl, add the almond flour and whisk to break up the lumps. Add the melted butter, vanilla, and sugar and mix with a spoon. Add a tiny drizzle of water, about 1–2 tablespoons as needed. Once the crust comes together when you squeeze it, it's ready.

Spray the silicon muffin pan (or regular muffin tin) with non-stick cooking spray. Wipe the top clean of the spray, so it doesn't burn in the oven.

Place the silicon muffin pan onto a baking sheet. Add 1 heaping tablespoon of almond flour crust into the bottom of the muffin pan or tin and press into the bottom. It will not go up the sides. It should be about ½-inch thickness. I bake 12 muffins at a time. Do it in 2 batches.

Bake the crust for 6–7 minutes until firm. Allow it to cool. Feel free to use any base for these cheesecakes.

Some other base options: animal crackers, graham crackers, gingersnaps, vanilla and cream cookies, chocolate and cream cookies, and gluten-free cookies. You can even pulse in some nuts if you wish. In this case, use a high-speed blender or food processor. Be creative. Pulse the cookies into a powder-like consistency, then add the butter, vanilla, sugar, and water as needed.

Note: The crust was not as crunchy in the silicone muffin holder. I did find it crisped better in the muffin tin. It was very easy to pop the cheesecakes out of the silicone holder, but if you are careful and use a butter knife to loosen the cheesecake in the tin, you should be able to get them out easily.

Prepare the Berry Sauce.

In a small pan, add the blackberries, blueberries, and a drizzle of water, about ⅛ of a cup. Allow this to boil and reduce. Smash the berries with the back of a wooden spoon. You may add a little sugar if you wish; I usually skip it, although a compote is made with sugar syrup and fresh fruit.

Strain the berries over a bowl to catch the berry juice. Set the berry juice aside to cool. Repeat the same process with the raspberries. Add the jam to the pan with the berries along with ⅛ cup more water and reduce. You can use some of the raspberry sauce to fully cover a few of

the mini cheesecakes for a decorative, visual appeal. This is what they do in a French bakery near me.

Make the Cheesecake Filling.

In a high-speed blender, add the cottage cheese, cream cheese, sour cream, powdered sugar, vanilla, lemon juice, and cornstarch. Blend using the agitator stick until smooth.

Note: I used a powdered sugar that contains tapioca starch. It works great in this recipe as a thickening agent, so I highly recommend using it, or you can add some tapioca starch to regular powdered sugar.

Spoon the cheesecake filling into the muffin cups. Don't go all the way to the top – leave a little room – but you can fill these up nicely. They will not overflow and will keep their shape since there is no egg in this recipe.

Bake in the oven at 325 degrees for about 22–25 minutes. They bake fast. Resist the urge to open the oven for around 20 minutes, then check them. They should be firm with a little jiggle. Repeat the process with the second batch. You should have enough filling for about 6–8 more mini cheesecakes.

Harvest tip: Frozen fruit is the next best option if you cannot find fresh fruit. They freeze soon after harvest to preserve their nutrients. Choosing wild blueberries over regular blueberries provides even more health benefits.

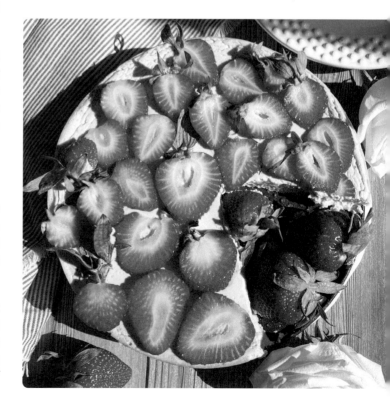

CHOCOLATE GLAZED
OAT-DATE ENERGY BITES
(Gluten Free)

These will be a great addition for healthy snacking for your family. Easy pop-and-go bites! It is an easily adaptable recipe that can be adjusted to your tastes. You can add roasted and salted sunflower and pumpkin seeds with a maple glaze, or just plain or change it up and add some crushed nuts instead, maybe walnuts or almonds. If you aren't a fan of tahini, substitute with some creamy almond butter. If you find the energy bite batter slightly wet, add an additional tablespoon of flax meal.

If you want to serve these as a beautiful dessert for your healthy guests, dip them in the melted and glossy chocolate. Be fancy and add some crushed food-grade rose petals. Instead, you can roll these in finely shredded coconut flakes or even crushed seeds.

INGREDIENTS:

- 10 pitted medjool dates, soaked in hot water and drained
- 1 cup gluten-free rolled oats, pulsed
- 2 tablespoons flax meal
- 3 tablespoons roasted and salted pumpkin and sunflower seeds, maple glazed (or substitute with crushed nuts)
- 3 tablespoons sugar-free maple syrup
- 2 tablespoons tahini (or creamy almond butter)
- 1 cup semi-sweet chocolate chips
- 1 teaspoon coconut oil
- Food-safe rose petals or finely shredded coconut or more crushed seeds (optional)
- High-speed blender (or food processor)
- Small pan

First, soak the dates in hot water for 10 minutes to soften. Then drain. Reserve a little liquid. Set these aside.

In a high-speed blender, add the oats and pulse for 1–2 minutes until broken down. Add the flax meal, sunflower, and pumpkin seeds. Continue to blend for an additional minute. Alternatively, you may use the food processor.

Add the mixture to a saucepan and heat until fragrant, about 5 minutes on low heat. This will give them a deep nutty flavor.

Add the softened dates to a clean blender with maple syrup. Pulse until they are broken down into bits. You may add 1 tablespoon of water from the drained dates if you need a little more liquid.

Note: Medjool dates have a sweet, caramel taste and chewy texture. They are a natural sweetener. If you prefer to avoid artificial sweeteners, use regular maple syrup in lieu of sugar-free maple syrup in recipes.

In a medium-sized bowl, combine the dates with the toasted flour-seed mixture. Swirl in the tahini until the dough is moistened. You should be able to easily roll into balls. I use a cookie scoop, about 1 ½ tablespoons. If they are too sticky, add 1 or more tablespoons of flax meal.

Prepare the Chocolate Glaze.

Baker's tip: Adding coconut oil to chocolate creates a glossy glaze.

Add the chocolate chips to a paper bowl. Add 1 teaspoon of coconut oil. Place in the microwave for 1 minute and stir. Heat another 30 seconds and stir to redistribute the heat and melt the remaining chips. If you overheat the chocolate, it will clump, so heat and then check every 30 seconds.

Using a tiny spoon, dip the bite into the chocolate to coat. Allow it to drip over the bowl and place onto a parchment-lined paper plate. Add the rose petals, finely shredded coconut, or crushed seeds. Place in the freezer for 10 minutes to harden. These will last in the fridge for up to 5 days or you may freeze (defrost before eating).

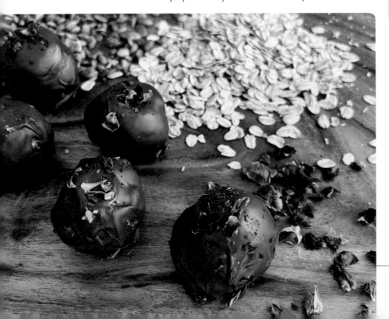

HEALTHY TRUFFLES
(Gluten Free)

INGREDIENTS:

- 9 regular-sized rice cakes, lightly salted
- ⅓ –½ cup melted mini semi-sweet chocolate chips
- ¾ cup super-fine almond flour
- 1 medium banana, mashed
- 2 tablespoons vanilla extract
- 2 tablespoons olive oil (or coconut oil)
- 1 tablespoon sugar-free maple syrup
- Water as needed
- Add ins: more chocolate chips, chopped nuts, seeds
- Coating: finely chopped nuts, melted chocolate, or cocoa powder
- High-speed blender

In a high-speed blender using the agitator stick, pulse the rice cakes into a powder-like consistency. Dump the pulsed rice cakes into a large bowl.

Next, melt the chocolate in a microwave-safe bowl for about 1 minute and 30 seconds and stir. Heat an additional 10–15 seconds until melted. Then set it aside.

Whisk the almond flour and add it to the bowl with the pulsed rice cakes and mix. Add the mashed banana, vanilla extract, olive oil, maple syrup, and mix. Lastly, add the melted chocolate and water as needed. You may add in some more chocolate chips, nuts, or seeds.

Make the balls and freeze for 20 minutes, then you can coat the balls with the coating of your choice: more melted chocolate, cocoa powder, crushed nuts, or leave plain. These balls freeze well.

These are a great healthy snack with coffee or tea.

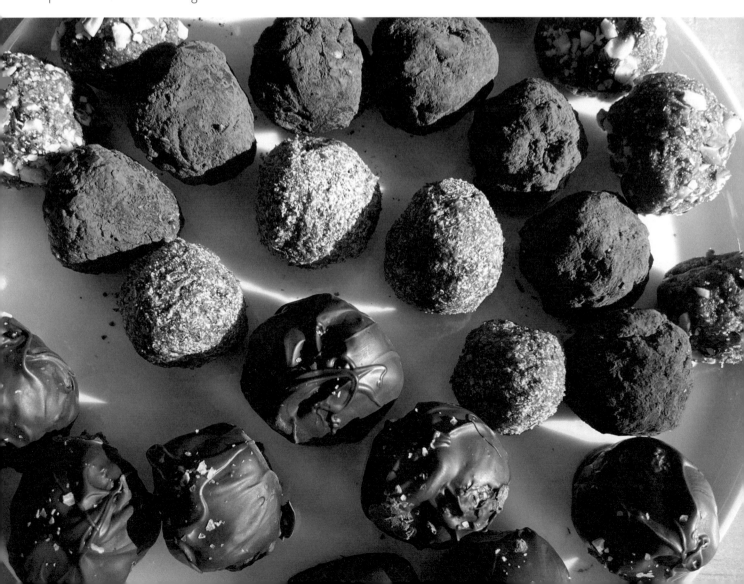

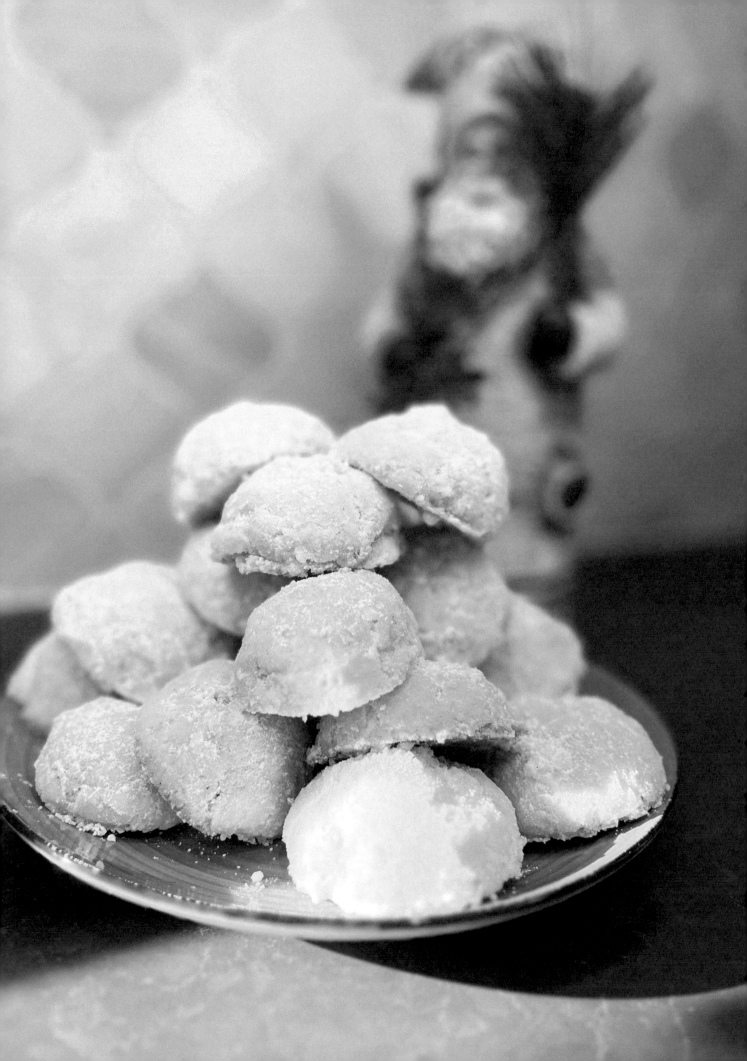

CARDAMOM-LAVENDER SNOWBALL COOKIES
(Gluten Free and Nut Free)

YIELDS 30 COOKIES

Everyone loves the ever-popular Mexican wedding cookies, also known as snowball cookies, that contain pecans, a nut my family does not eat. I used to make a version of these for Jack. These are a gluten-free and nut-free cookie, but you can swap out the gluten-free flour for regular flour and add some chopped pecans if you wish. The combination of aromatic spices and crushed herbs make this a truly irresistible multi-sensory experience. The butter is added to keep that quintessential crumble you'd expect from this cookie. They are a great gift-giving idea during the holidays.

INGREDIENTS:

- 2 tablespoons Lavender Simple Syrup (recipe follows)
- ½ teaspoon cardamom
- ½ teaspoon dried rosemary
- ½ teaspoon food-safe dried lavender flowers
- 2 sticks salted butter, softened
- 1 cup powdered sugar (or confectioner's sugar)
- 2 tablespoons cream cheese, room temperature
- 2 cups gluten-free flour (I used King Arthur Baking Company's Measure for Measure Gluten-Free Flour), spooned and leveled
- Powdered sugar for rolling cookie balls
- Mortar and pestle
- Stand mixer with paddle attachment

Preheat the oven to 350 degrees.

Make the Lavender Simple Syrup.

In a small pot, stir together equal parts water and sugar. Bring to a boil, stir, and let the sugar dissolve. Stir until translucent. This creates the simple syrup, then you can infuse flavor. Take it off the burner, add in the lavender flowers, give it a quick stir, and cover. Let steep until it's cool. Strain, and discard flowers. Then refrigerate until ready to use. Use this to infuse flavor into cocktails, cakes, or cookies. Store in an air-tight container in the refrigerator for 1–2 weeks. You can use other garden herbs like thyme, rosemary, or mint too.

Note: Use fragrant English lavender. This is culinary lavender and is available at farmer's markets, or online. I harvest the lavender from my garden in the summer, dry it, and jar it for use during the year and for this delicious loaf. Alternatively, you can buy lavender simple syrup.

Add the cardamom, dried rosemary, and dried lavender flowers to the mortar and pestle and grind them down until all the rosemary and lavender flowers are broken into bits. Set this aside.

In the bowl of the stand mixer, add the butter and mix until smooth. Combine with confectioner's sugar and mix on medium speed for 2 minutes. Add the cream cheese, lavender simple syrup, and spices. Mix on medium speed until well combined.

In a separate bowl, add flour and whisk. Slowly add the flour to the stand mixer bowl with the wet ingredients and mix on medium speed until the dough starts to form together. If it's a little wet, add one tablespoon at a time of flour until the dough is no longer sticky.

Prepare 2 baking sheets lined with parchment paper. Roll cookie dough into 1-inch balls and place onto baking sheet.

Bake cookies for 15–17 minutes, until slightly browned on the bottom. Allow cookies to sit on baking sheet for a few minutes, then roll in powdered sugar twice.

I have also rolled the cookie dough ball into powdered sugar and then baked them. In this case the cookies will take closer to 17 minutes. Once slightly cooled, roll them twice in a fresh batch of powdered sugar.

These freeze well. One of my all-time favorite cookies!

HEALTHY MAGIC COOKIE BARS
(Gluten Free)

Magic Cookie Bars are known for their graham cracker crust base and for using condensed milk, that's why they are so sweet. The challenge was to make a slightly healthier crust as well as make it gluten free. I also wanted to avoid butter. It's a great pick-me-up or mid-afternoon treat with coffee. These are best chilled in the fridge.

INGREDIENTS:

Almond Cookie Base:

- 4 cups super-fine almond flour, spooned and leveled
- 1 cup tahini
- ½ cup light brown sugar
- 2 tablespoon olive oil
- ¼ cup water
- 9x13-inch pan

Top Layer:

- 12 large medjool dates, pitted
- 1 cup water
- ½ cup sugar-free maple syrup
- 1 cup creamy almond butter, salted
- Medium-sized pot

Toppings:

- ½ cup chopped roasted and salted almonds
- ½ cup shredded coconut
- ½ cup semi-sweet mini chocolate chips

Preheat the oven to 350 degrees.

In a medium-sized bowl, whisk the flour. Add the tahini, brown sugar, water, and olive oil. Mix with clean hands. If it's a little dry, add more oil a tiny drizzle at a time. Once it forms into a dough, press it into a parchment lined pan.

Bake at 350 degrees for 6 minutes or until somewhat firm.

In a small pot, gently boil the dates in 1 cup water. Once softened, allow them to cool. Strain out liquid. (You can use the liquid for my Dogels (page 5)

Leave the dates in the pot and gently mash. Next, add the maple syrup and almond butter. Heat on low. Mix until well combined, then take the mixture off the heat. You'll want to work with the mixture while it's warm.

Once the base layer has cooled a little, press the top layer (date-almond mixture) onto the bottom layer with your hands, covering the entire base.

Next, press in the chopped nuts, shredded coconut, and last the chocolate chips.

Place in the fridge to solidify for 1 hour. Then cut into squares and enjoy!

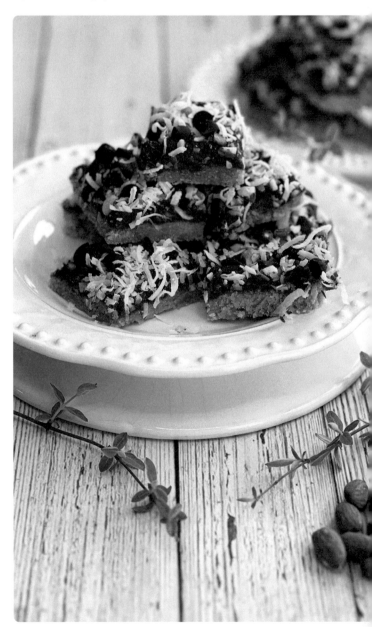

HEALTHY BROWNIE BITES

They are so fudgy, and there is no presence of black beans, applesauce, or dates. Feel free to add some finely chopped walnuts and experiment using a milk chocolate cocoa powder which will give these a lighter color.

INGREDIENTS:

- 1 (29-ounce) can black beans (use only 2 cups), rinsed and drained
- 5 large medjool dates (pitted), soaked in hot water and drained
- ½ cup applesauce (or pumpkin purée)
- ¾ cup light brown sugar, packed
- 2 tablespoon cooled coffee (optional)
- 1 teaspoon vanilla
- 1 egg yolk, room temperature
- ½ cup all-purpose flour, spooned and leveled (or whole wheat flour)
- ¼ cup special dark chocolate cocoa powder, spooned and leveled
- 2 level tablespoons flax meal
- ½ teaspoon baking soda
- ½ cup large semi-sweet chocolate chips, melted
- ¼ cup semi-sweet mini chocolate chips (or chopped dark chocolate bar)
- A sprinkle of sea salt (optional)
- Mini muffin tin
- Non-stick cooking spray
- High-speed blender (or food processor)
- Stand mixer with paddle attachment

Preheat the oven to 350 degrees.

Rinse and thoroughly drain the black beans. Add the beans to the blender and pulse using the agitator stick until smooth, about 1 minute. You may see some bits of beans. Drain the dates and finely chop them into tiny pieces. Set these aside.

In the bowl of the stand mixer, add the bean mixture, chopped dates, applesauce (or pumpkin purée), brown sugar, cooled coffee, and vanilla. Mix to combine on medium-low speed. Last, stream in the premixed egg yolk and mix on low until it is combined, about 30 seconds.

In a medium-sized bowl, add the flour, cocoa powder, flax meal, and baking soda. Be sure to spoon and level the cocoa powder especially. If you scoop it up, you will end up with too much, making these brownies very dry. Whisk to combine.

Note: I have not experimented with gluten-free flour, but feel free to substitute the flour with gluten-free flour. Also, you may swap out the all-purpose flour for whole wheat flour for a healthier alternative.

Add the dry ingredients to the wet ingredients and mix on medium-low speed. Add the slightly cooled melted chocolate and fold the chocolate chips into the brownie batter.

Spray the mini muffin tin with non-stick cooking spray. Add 1 heaping tablespoon of brownie batter for each muffin.

Bake for roughly 16 minutes. Take one out at 16 minutes and break it open. It should be very fudgy, and that means it's baked long enough. You don't want to dry these out.

Take the muffins out of the tin by gently loosening with a knife and place onto a cooling rack. These are best served after a few hours of sitting at room temperature and even better on day 2. Refrigerate leftovers for up to 5 days or freeze.

At Christmastime, make a double batch of these black bean brownies and spread the batter onto 2 small parchment-lined baking sheets. Bake in the oven until cooked through and allow them to cool. Then make a light icing with a combination of powdered sugar and water. Pour over each cake layer to further sweeten them.

Top one layer with a raspberry or strawberry jam. Flip the other cake pan on top of the jam-layered cake, pull off the parchment paper. Once this has completely cooled, add a chocolate ganache and swirl in some melted white chocolate. Let it set in the fridge.

This was my version of the ever-popular Venetian cakes minus all the food dye, and mine is a 2-layered cake.

Chocolate ganache is simply melted chocolate with heavy whipping cream. Melt chocolate in a heat-safe bowl over a pot of hot water. Temper the whipped cream slowly, whisking continuously. Pour over the cake once slightly cooled.

Let it set in the fridge overnight and cut into squares. Cut and clean the knife after each cut. Undeniably delicious, and you cannot detect the black beans whatsoever. Refrigerate leftovers for up to 5 days or freeze.

CARROT CAKE

While recipe testing these cupcakes, the memories came flooding back to me. I was an aerobics instructor in high school and taught for nearly a decade. I would pack the classes up to 100-plus people. It was really something to see and hear, as the ladies in this all-women fitness center loved to belt it out and have fun. I recall, fondly, getting a slice of carrot cake after class with one of my fellow teachers. The cake was so delicious and creamy, and I savored every bite, especially the walnuts.

Life has changed for me now that my husband and son are allergic to nuts, so making carrot cake filled with walnuts is not an option for my family, but I have always loved carrot cake, especially paired with a cream cheese icing. This recipe does not contain nuts, but you can add a ½ cup of chopped walnuts. The addition of applesauce, sour cream, and mascarpone cheese make this cake so creamy.

INGREDIENTS:

- 2 cups finely grated organic carrots, roughly 6 carrots
- 2 cups cake flour, spooned and leveled
- ¾ cup granulated sugar
- ½ cup light brown sugar, packed
- ½ cup light sour cream
- ½ cup unsweetened applesauce (or finely chopped pineapple plus juices)
- 2 heaping tablespoons mascarpone cheese (or cream cheese)
- ¾ cup extra virgin olive oil
- 2 large eggs
- 1 teaspoon baking soda
- 1 teaspoon baking powder
- 1 ½ teaspoons cinnamon
- 1 teaspoon ground ginger
- ½ teaspoon freshly grated ginger
- 1 teaspoon vanilla extract
- Tiny pinch nutmeg
- ⅛ teaspoon table salt
- ¾ cup chopped walnuts (optional)
- 2 (8-inch) round pans or muffin tins with tulip liners
- Stand mixer with paddle attachment
- High-speed blender (optional)

Cinnamon-Ginger Cream Cheese Icing:

- 3 ½ cups powdered sugar
- 1 teaspoon clear vanilla extract
- 1 stick salted butter, softened
- 8 ounces cream cheese, softened
- Tiny dash cinnamon and ginger
- Stand mixer with whisk attachment

Preheat the oven to 350 degrees.

If you are making a double layer cake, butter the sides of the pans and lightly dust them with all-purpose flour, be thorough. Cut a circle of parchment paper for the bottom of can pan so the cake doesn't stick. If you are preparing a muffin pan, use the tulip liners. This recipe will yield 15 large cupcakes.

First, rinse, dry, and peel the carrots. You have two options. You can finely grate the carrots, albeit this is tedious. Alternatively, rough chop the carrots and add them to the high-speed blender or an electric vegetable chopper to chop into fine bits. I found this way is the easiest and worked great. Then measure roughly 2 cups and set these aside.

In a bowl, whisk together the flour, baking powder, baking soda, cinnamon, ground ginger, nutmeg, and salt.

In the stand mixer bowl, add the sugar, oil, sour cream, applesauce, mascarpone, freshly grated ginger, and vanilla. Mix on medium-high speed until fully combined. Next, premix the eggs and stream into the mixer bowl. Mix on medium-high speed to fully combine ingredients. Scrape down the sides and bottom of the bowl with a spatula to be sure all the ingredients are well combined.

Add the dry ingredients to the wet ingredients in 2 stages. Mix until the ingredients are smooth. Then add the chunky ingredients—carrots and walnuts (if adding)—and mix with a rubber spatula to combine (or keep on low speed in the stand mixer).

Pour the batter into the cake pan and tap on the counter to level out. Alternatively, spoon into the cupcake liners.

Allergy note: If you are concerned with allergies but would like a few cupcakes with nuts. Do not add the walnuts when you add the carrots. Add the walnuts after

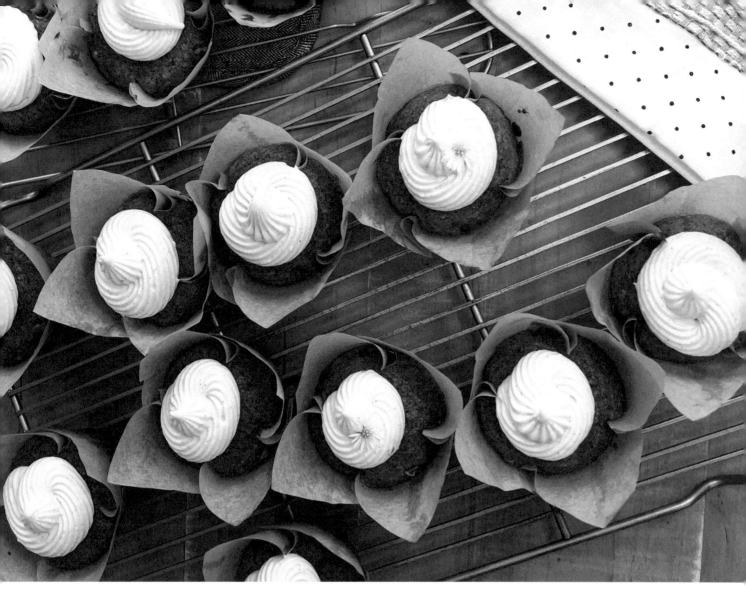

you spoon the cake batter into the cupcake liners, and gently mix with a spoon to combine. It's best to use a different color liner in this case, to denote the cupcakes containing nuts from those that do not have any—write it down so you remember!

Place in the oven and bake at 350 degrees for roughly 45 minutes, or until the cupcakes or cake are firm to the touch and a golden brown. Cupcakes will bake in roughly 30 minutes, turn halfway.

Make the Icing.

In the stand mixer bowl with whish attachment, add the softened butter. Alternatively, you can use the hand mixer. Add the cream cheese and beat on medium speed until light and fluffy, about 2 minutes. Gradually add the sugar: Stop the mixer and scrape down the sides and bottom of bowl with a rubber spatula. Add 1 cup powdered sugar at a time. Return to medium speed. Repeat scraping and beating in the remaining powdered sugar.

Note: For the cupcakes you will only need roughly 3 cups of powdered sugar.

Add the vanilla, a tiny dash of both cinnamon and ginger. For a whiter icing, use only a tiny dash of cinnamon and ginger and a clear vanilla extract. Go very light on the cinnamon or skip altogether. Beat the frosting again on medium speed until smooth and creamy. As always, taste it to be sure the flavors are well balanced. If it's too sweet, add 1 tablespoon of cream cheese.

Baker's tip: If serving adults, feel free to add in a little rum into the icing. You can even infuse some into the cake.

Icing storage: If not using the icing immediately, the cream cheese frosting can be refrigerated for up to 2 to 3 days in an airtight container. Before using, bring to room temperature and then beat until smooth.

Store iced cake or cupcakes in an air-tight container for 4 days in fridge.

HEALTHY LIFESTYLE TIPS

BY

SAMARA KRAFT
MS, RDN, CDCES

Me: What is the gut microbiome and why is it important?

Samara: The gut microbiome is a collection of microorganisms that live together in our digestive tract and have an effect on our health. There are different types of microorganisms such as bacteria, fungi, viruses, parasites, and other microorganisms which can be both helpful and potentially harmful. In a healthy gut there is a balance of all these. Problems may arise when there is an imbalance between the healthy and unhealthy microorganisms caused by infections, disease, certain diets, and prolonged use of antibiotics.

The gut microbiome is initially determined by genetics, but later is influenced by our environment, diet, and overall lifestyle. A well-balanced, healthy gut can decrease inflammation, alleviate constipation, improve immunity, improve bone health through enhanced calcium absorption, optimize blood glucose control, benefit mental health, and promote weight loss. It is important to prioritize our gut health.

Me: How do we improve our gut health and reduce inflammation. Do you recommend any particular diets? Are there certain foods we should avoid?

A Mediterranean-style diet including plenty of fruit, vegetables, whole grain breads and other grains, potatoes, legumes, nuts, seeds, olive oil, dairy products, eggs, fish, and poultry is beneficial to gut health. I suggest replacing saturated fats, trans fats, and hydrogenated oils as well as eliminating processed foods like luncheon meats, sugary foods and drinks, and fried foods. This will further aid in decreasing inflammation and improving one's overall gut health.

Me: What's the difference between probiotic and prebiotic?

Samara: Probiotics are live bacteria and yeasts that are found in various types of food or taken through supplements. Probiotics in the body are referred to as "good" or "helpful" bacteria and yeasts and can promote a healthy gut.

Prebiotics are indigestible fibers found in plants that act as food for the good bacteria and probiotics found in the digestive tract. After prebiotics are consumed, they are digested and travel to the colon where they are fermented and metabolized in the microbiome.

Me: Probiotic and prebiotic powders and supplements are very popular. For those who do not want to take these powders and supplements, what foods will most benefit our gut health? Are fermented foods good for gut health?

Samara: It is always best to try to get probiotics and prebiotics through diet in order to take advantage of other beneficial elements that food can provide. Food that contains probiotics and prebiotics often include vitamins, minerals, and phytochemicals, which additionally have many health benefits.

Probiotics are found naturally in many foods. Many fermented foods contain live cultures that increase the good, healthy bacteria, or probiotics in the gut microbiome. Some examples which are the most beneficial to the gut microbiome include yogurt, kefir, cottage cheese, sauerkraut, kimchi, kombucha, traditional buttermilk, some types of sour cream, feta, provolone, and parmesan cheese. It's important to note that not all fermented foods are good sources of probiotics. Processing and using heating techniques for canning can affect the availability of probiotics.

Good sources of prebiotics include pistachios, almonds, onions, leeks, garlic, tomatoes, cocoa, flaxseeds, chai and zen basil seeds, konjac, legumes, oats, bran, barley, chick peas, red kidney beans, soybeans, whole grains, fruit such as apples, bananas, grapefruit, watermelon, and green leafy vegetables. Sometimes bread, yogurt, and cereals are fortified with prebiotics.

Powders and supplements are sometimes the only option in order to increase prebiotic and probiotic consumption for people who have difficulty with digestion or have gastrointestinal conditions.

Me: Alzheimer's and dementia are affecting more and more of our aging population. Although there is no single cause according to research, it is suggested that there are multiple factors at work like: age, genetics, and lifestyle. The risk of developing Alzheimer's as you age appears to be increased by many conditions that damage the heart and blood vessels. These include heart disease, diabetes, stroke, high blood pressure, and high cholesterol. Can you explain this further?

Samara: A healthy lifestyle filled with exercise and healthy diet may decrease the risk of dementia. Obesity, elevated cholesterol levels, hypertension, diabetes, inactivity, and smoking are huge risk factors for developing dementia. All these vascular diseases, such as diabetes, stroke, hypertension, and high cholesterol can increase your risk of heart disease, as well. However, you do have some control. Overall lifestyle has a huge influence on heart and brain health. Eating lots of colorful vegetables, fruit, legumes, whole grains, and limiting saturated, trans fats, added sugars, and alcohol all can contribute to a healthy heart and in turn may decrease the risk of dementia.

Me: What foods specifically will get our brain to function at an optimal level?

Samara: Diet and lifestyle play a huge role in our cognitive health, similar to the diet to help with heart health. Eating a diet that is abundant in fruit, vegetables, legumes, whole grains, protein sources from plants, and fish keeps our brain functioning at an optimal level. Make sure to avoid saturated and trans fats, sugary drinks, fried foods, and limit refined grains.

Heart-healthy food is also the best brain food. Not only does spinach keep you strong, but it also helps with cognition, along with other greens such as kale, collard greens, and broccoli. These foods contain phylloquinone, lutein, and folate which are thought to be responsible for slowing down memory decline. Aim to get at least one serving of these foods into your diet per day in order to take advantage of these benefits.

The following components of food are influential to our brain health:

- *Foods that are high in omega-3 fatty acids help with cognition by sharpening signals in the brain and correspond to a level of beta-amyloid, the protein found in the brain of those with Alzheimer's disease. Good sources of omega-3 fatty acids include fatty fish such as salmon, cod, mackerel, and tuna. Omega-3 fatty acids are also found in flaxseed, krill, chia, kiwi, butternuts, and walnuts.*

- *Flavonoids are phytochemical compounds responsible for bright colors found in plants and they can help with improving memory. Flavonoids are found in berries, cherries, apples, oils, soybeans, citrus fruit, cocoa, coffee, green tea, ginkgo tree, and red wine.*

- *Vitamin B6 and Vitamin B12 (folate) help preserve cognition. Great sources of Vitamin B6 include canned chick peas, tahini, sockeye salmon, chicken breast, beef liver, and even breakfast cereals that are fortified. Vitamin B12 is found in fish, meat, poultry, eggs, milk, beef liver and clams, and fortified foods such as cereal and nutritional yeasts.*

- *Vitamin D, abundantly found in mushrooms, fatty fish, and fortified products such as milk, breads, and cereals, help to preserve brain function. Of course, going outside and catching some sun for 15 minutes or longer is an excellent source, as well.*

- *Vitamin E also helps with cognition. Great sources of Vitamin E are asparagus, avocado, nuts, olives, peanuts, seeds, spinach, vegetable oil, and wheat germ.*

- *Choline is another nutrient that enhances brain function. Great sources of choline are egg yolks, chicken, veal, turkey, lettuce, and liver.*

- *Saturated and trans fatty acids have been shown to decrease brain function. Reduce your intake of whole milk products, lard, butter, margarine, coconut oil, palm and palm kernel oil.*

- *Exercise and healthy lifestyle habits such as getting adequate sleep, being mentally stimulated, limiting (or avoiding) alcohol, drugs and caffeine, maintaining a healthy weight, being social, and drinking adequate water for proper hydration, are shown to positively influence brain health.*

Me: Let's talk further about a heart healthy diet and lifestyle changes that will impact our heart health. This is an area I take very seriously given the fact that both of my parents had heart disease.

Samara: The leading cause of death in the world is known to be heart disease. The American Heart Association suggests that lifestyle and diet are helpful in protecting the heart. Eating a diet made up of a variety of fruit and vegetables, whole grains, low-fat or nonfat dairy, plant source proteins such as legumes and nuts, fiber, and lean animal products, and liquid nontropical vegetable oils such as olive, canola, corn, peanut, safflower, soybean, and sunflower oils can help heart health. In addition, minimizing processed food, added sugars and salt, limiting alcohol, and avoiding smoking are influential towards heart health. Being at an optimal weight and knowing your calorie needs and avoiding consuming more than you are expending is recommended.

Being physically active, aiming weekly for at least 150 minutes of moderate physical activity or 75 minutes of vigorous activity is important for prevention and management of heart disease.

Me: Do you recommend doing annual physicals to identify high sugar or high cholesterol? Can you be thin and have high cholesterol?

Samara: Going to your doctor annually is helpful in monitoring your health. There are health conditions that are silent, which makes it only possible to provide a diagnosis through bloodwork. For example, many people live for years while unknowingly having diabetes. If they had learned about their diagnosis earlier on, through a routine medical office visit, they may have been able to implement lifestyle changes to prevent from developing full-blown diabetes.

Very often being overweight causes stress and burden on the body, causing it to work much harder to be efficient. However, genetics also play a huge role in one's health. You most definitely can be thin and have elevated cholesterol, hypertension, diabetes, and many other medical conditions due to your genetic makeup, so it's important to have an annual visit to your doctor.

Me: How can we possibly fend off the early onset of diabetes as we age? Identifying it early through routine physical exams and bloodwork is important. What are some dietary changes we can make?

Samara: Being at a desirable weight for height can help reduce chances of developing diabetes as we age. The risk of developing diabetes can be decreased by making healthy lifestyle choices, being physically active, following a low-fat diet made up of lots of vegetables and fruit, avoiding added sugars and unhealthy fats, and not exceeding individualized calorie needs. Although there is a genetic element to diabetes, obesity can also increase the risk of developing diabetes since the body has to work much harder to function, which can lead to prediabetes and diabetes.

Me: What do you think the leading cause of obesity is in our country?

Samara: Obesity is caused by poor lifestyle habits. This includes a lack of physical activity, sedentary lifestyle, inadequate sleep, and unhealthy diet. Processed foods, portion sizes, calorie dense foods made up of unhealthy fats and added sugars are to blame for consuming excessive calories, which leads to obesity.

Me: Does portion size matter? What is a good rule of thumb for pasta, rice, or any carbohydrates? Do you think Europeans are generally thinner due to better portion control?

Samara: Portion size of food has grown over the years. It started increasing in the 1970s and drastically increased in the 1980s, continuing throughout the years since then. Simultaneously, the rate of obesity has increased over the years and serving sizes listed on packages have been following the average weight of our population. This is just a hint about how our portions sizes have been changing over the past 50 years. Even our dinner plates have increased in size.

Portion control is very important in providing a well-rounded, healthy diet, which in turn may decrease the risk of developing certain chronic diseases that are related to excessive body weight. Try eating off of a smaller plate to help control portions. A good technique to control portions is by visually sectioning off your plate to consist of half of the plate being made up of non-starchy vegetables, a quarter of the plate should contain lean proteins, and the last quarter could be healthy, high-fiber carbohydrates.

Me: Do collagen supplements make a difference in hair, skin, nail, and bone health?

Samara: Collagen, a protein made up of amino acids found in muscle, connective tissue, tendons, and bones, is quite abundant in animals and in our body. As we age, collagen decreases, causing a change in the appearance of skin and it also affects bone health.

Diet and lifestyle play a role in the collagen in our body. Eating a diet with adequate amounts of lean protein (chicken, fish, and legumes) intake along with other nutritional components, such as antioxidants from plant compounds, vitamin C rich foods (oranges, strawberries, pineapple, mango, kiwi, peppers, and broccoli), calcium, vitamin D, and zinc, enable the body to create and support the collagen already in our body that is needed for glowing skin and bone health.

Collagen supplements have been shown to be safe and may sometimes contain added protein which may be helpful. However, sometimes the manufacturers put other ingredients in the supplement, such as herbs and large amounts of vitamins, which can cause other side effects. It is important to note that eating a diet high in processed foods, added sugars, and fried foods can also negatively affect collagen in the body. Eating a lean, unprocessed healthy diet, avoiding smoking, and limiting alcohol can support our collagen health.

Me: Can you explain intermittent fasting?

Samara: Intermittent fasting (IF) is a diet based on a specific patterned eating schedule that can help promote weight loss. IF patterns range from either restricting eating during certain hours of the day or limiting the number of calories consumed per day. Common patterns of IF include eating over 8 hours and fasting the remaining 16 hours of the day or eating over 10 hours and fasting the remaining 14 hours of the day, or alternate day fasting with any of the above. The important thing is that food is consumed on a scheduled pattern. Think of it like an appetite reset.

The results of IF can be weight loss due to decreased eating hours, which contribute to less calories consumed over the course of the day and burning fat after the daily consumed and required calories are utilized. However, it is still important to make sure that, during eating hours food choices and portion sizes are mindful and intentional. In addition to weight loss, intermittent fasting can create a leaner body, may decrease the risk of chronic disease, and help with clearer thinking. Although IF can have positive results for some, it is not recommended for children, those with certain chronic diseases, and pregnant and nursing women.

In summary, optimizing your health is a multi-pronged, balanced approach. Eating a diet filled with healthy, nutrient-rich foods, being mindful with food choices, practicing portion control, exercising daily, and getting proper amounts of rest are the key to living a healthy lifestyle. It is also important to listen to your body's needs and to eat and enjoy the food that you love.

NOURISH has plenty of healthy recipes and meal options, along with helpful nutritional tips. Eating a healthy diet made up of healthy home cooked meals that focus on legumes, fish, vegetables, and fruit with the addition of lean cuts of meat will help you achieve your best health. Enjoying the foods that you love like cakes, cookies, and homemade bread is fine, in moderation. It's about finding that balance.

> *Disclaimer: This Q & A does not recommend any one specific diet, but is educating you on dietary trends, eating, and other nutrition related health risks. As always, consult with your medical provider regarding any medical concerns, or taking supplements. There may be some contraindications for some groups regarding eating some types of mushrooms. Consulting with a Registered Dietitian Nutritionist (RDN), a credentialed healthcare food and nutrition expert, is a great way to get a full picture of your nutritional needs based off evidence-based information, your individual lifestyle, and nutritional goals. Nutritional needs are based on age, gender, medical history, and individualized goals.*

Works Cited :

Coleman Collins MS, RDN, LD, Sherry. "Entering the World of Prebiotics - Are they a precursor to Good Gut Health?" *Today's Dietitian*, vol. 16, no. 12, Dec. 2014, p.12, www.todaysdietitian.com/newarchives/120914p12.shtml.

Zhao PhD, Liping and Lam PhD, Yan Y. "The Microbiome and Digestive Health: A Look at Prebiotics." 2nd part; (4 part CME series), 29 July 2019.

Villines, Zawn. "What is the difference between prebiotics and probiotics?" Medically reviewed by Westphalen, Dena. *Pharm D, Medical News Today*, 29 Oct 2018.

Morris MC, et al. "Nutrients and bioactive in green leafy vegetables and cognitive decline." *Neurology, PubMed*, 16 Jan.

2018, www.pubmed.ncbi.nlm.nih.gov/29263222.

"Eating fish, chicken, nuts may lower risk of Alzheimer's disease." *Neurology*, 2 May 2012, www.eurekalert.org/news-releases/489917.

Gomez-Pinilla, Fernando. "Brain foods: the effects of nutrients on brain function." *Nature Reviews Neuroscience*, vol. 9, pp 568-578, July 2008, www.nature.com/articles/nrn2421.

"Leading Causes of Death." *National Center for Health Statistics*. Reviewed 6 Sept. 2022, www.cdc.gov/nchs/fastats/leading-causes-of-death.htm.

"Top 10 Causes of Death." *World Health Organization*. Dec. 2020, www.who.int/news-room/fact-sheets/detail/the-top-10-causes-of-death.

"The American Heart Association Diet and Lifestyle Recommendations." *American Heart Association*. Reviewed 1 Nov. 2021, www.heart.org/en/healthy-living/healthy-eating/eat-smart/nutrition-basics/aha-diet-and-lifestyle-recommendations.

Choi, Franchesca D., Sung, Calvin T., Juhasz, Margit L.W., Atanaskova Mesinkovsk, Natasha. "Oral Collagen Supplementation: A Systematic Review of Dermatological Applications." *PMID*. 306 81778. *J Drugs Dermatol. PubMed*, 1 Jan. 2019, www.pubmed.ncbi.nlm.nih.gov/30681787/.

Cabo Ph. D., Rafael and Mattson Ph.D., Mark. "Effects of Intermittent Fasting on Health, Aging and Disease." *N Engl J Med*, vol. 381, pp 2541-2551, 26 Dec. 2019, https://www.nejm.org/doi/full/10.1056/nejmra1905136.

Kubal MS, RD, Jillian."What is Collagen, and What is it good for?" *Healthline - Nutrition*, www.healthline.com/nutrition/collagen.

Klemm RDN, CD, LDN, Sarah. "Prebiotics and Probiotics: Creating a Healthier You." *American Academy of Nutrition and Dietetics*, Published 20 Jan. 2022, Reviewed Dec. 2021, www.eatright.org/food/vitamins-and-supplements/nutrient-rich-foods/prebiotics-and-probiotics-creating-a-healthier-you.

Erdmann, Jeanne. "What's the Difference Between Prebiotics and Probiotics?" *Discover Magazine*, 11 May 2021, www.discovermagazine.com/health/whats-the-difference-between-prebiotics-and-probiotics.

"What are Prebiotics and What Do They Do? Here's why prebiotics matter." *Cleveland Clinic healthessentials*, 14 March 2022, www.health.clevelandclinic.org/what-are-prebiotics/.

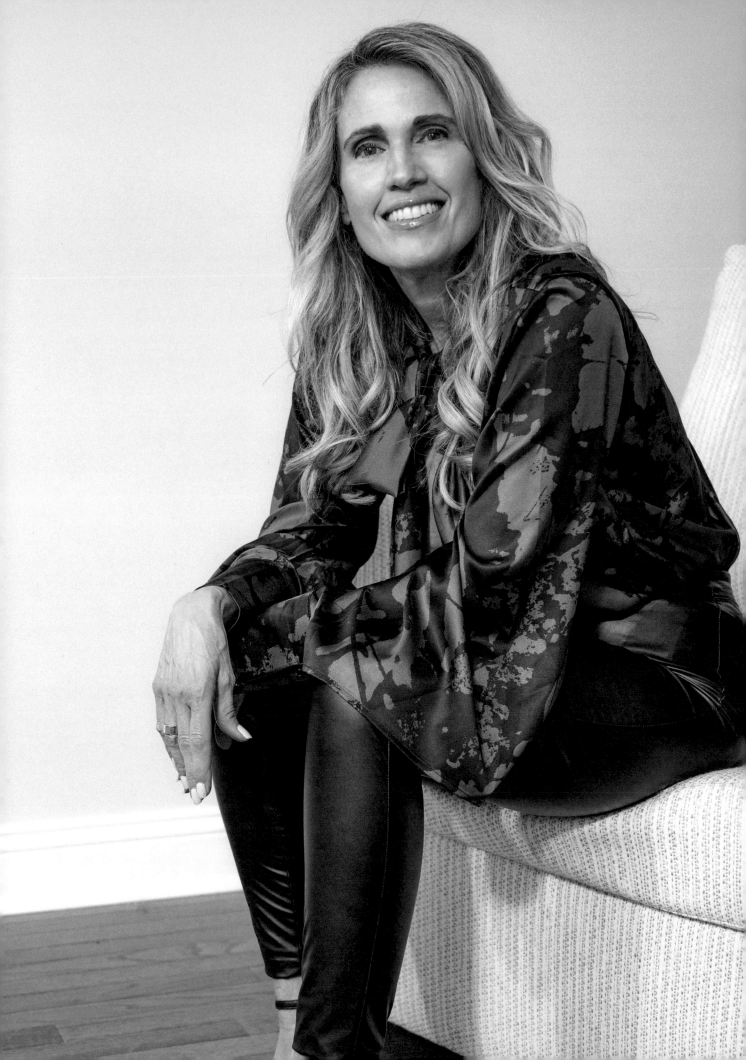

ABOUT THE AUTHOR

MARY ABITANTO is a prolific author, a professional food writer and food photographer, and an entrepreneur promoting her brand "Mariooch's Kitchen." She lives amidst horse and fresh produce farms in a scenic suburban town in New Jersey with her husband Peter, their children Maggie, Sydney, and Jack, and pups Charlie and Teddy. Mary is a talented self-taught chef and accomplished food stylist and food photographer, whose work has appeared in multiple magazines. Mariooch, "little Mary" in Italian, was a fitting choice for her brand as it was a nickname given to her by her Italian Father.

Mary pays tribute to her Italian roots in her cookbook, *Food That Will Gather Your Family*. She meticulously adapts recipes to preserve old-world flavor and heritage while updating recipes to fit her family's taste and healthy lifestyle. "Guard, honor, and cherish the family dinner," is her motto.

She also loves exploring other cultures in her cookbook, *Food From My Heart & Home*. It offers many healthy recipes with creative twists and is jam-packed with entertaining tips and styling ideas.

Gather For The Holidays has something for everybody and showcases Mary's talent for hosting large gatherings with well-planned menus and desserts that leave nothing to be desired. This book teaches you to create holiday magic for your guests.

NOURISH ~ Celebrating Nature's Harvest & A Healthy Lifestyle highlights Mary's passion for living a healthy lifestyle through good nutrition. She teaches you how to eat to maintain maximum nutrition and operate at optimal levels for sustained energy. This book will become a wonderful resource for living a healthy lifestyle.

Prior to turning her attention full-time to growing her brand, Mary earned her MBA. When she's not busy cooking, entertaining, or writing on her blog, she enjoys long walks and beach getaways. Her hidden talent is hitting the speed bag, which she considers akin to life, and says, "Timing is everything."

ABOUT THE AUTHOR

SAMARA KRAFT MS, RDN, CDCES, a former professional ballet dancer, has been practicing nutrition for over two decades and maintains a Master of Science degree in Clinical Nutrition and Dietetics from New York University. She owns and operates a private Clinical Nutrition practice where she counsels all different age groups on a wide array of diseases from diabetes to heart-related issues. She has been successful in helping her clients live healthy lifestyles over the past 2 decades.

She is also credentialed as a Certified Diabetes Care and Education Specialist through the National Certification Board for Diabetes Educators. She provides nutritional support and daily living tips to family members and her patients. She also specializes in cardiovascular disease management and prevention, metabolic syndrome, diabetes, insulin pump training, and weight management. She has become a trusted resource for her clients and family.

Samara lives in the beautiful suburbs of New Jersey with her husband Daniel and children Zachary, Maddox, and Chloe and four Siamese cats. She is a health and wellness advocate and nutritional specialist who enjoys doing Pilates, going to the ballet, and cooking healthy meals for her family. She also loves to travel around the world experiencing different cultures and cuisines.

HARVEST INDEX

A.

Apples
Baked Oatmeal with Apples, 11

Applesauce
Carrot Cake, 132
Healthy Brownie Bites, 131

Artichokes
Eggless Caesar Salad with Artichokes and Hearts of Palm, 53
Mezze Platter, 36

Arugula
Breaded Chicken Cutlets with Prosciutto, 91

Avocado
Broccomole, 40

B.

Banana
Green Matcha Shake, 8
Healthy Truffles, 127

Basil
Healthy Eggplant Parmesan, 65
Mushroom Ragu with Pappardelle, 98
Pasta Nerano, 103
Pesto, 105

Broccoli
Broccoli Pizza Crust, 111
Broccomole, 40

Beans, Black Beans
Black Bean and Sweet Potato Chili, 89
Healthy Brownie Bites, 131
Quinoa and Black Bean Bake, 39

Beans, White Beans (Cannellini)
Pasta Fagioli, 84

Blackberries
Blueberry-Blackberry Sauce, 124

Blueberries
Coffee Cake with Blueberries, 3
Blueberry-Blackberry Sauce, 124

Butternut Squash
Butternut Squash Soup, 55

C.

Cabbage
Collard Green Veggie Wraps with Seared Tofu, 76

Carrots
Black Bean and Sweet Potato Chili, 89
Beef Bourguignon, 87
Carrot Cake, 132
Carrot Fritters, 72
Collard Green Veggie Wraps with Seared Tofu, 76
Crudité Platter, 45
Mushroom Ragu with Pappardelle, 98
Pasta Fagioli, 84
Red Lentil Bolognese with Creamy Polenta, 100

Cauliflower
Cauliflower Pizza Crust, 115
Creamy Cauliflower Soup, 54
Crudité Platter, 45
Spicy Asian-Inspired Cauliflower Bites, 61

Celery
Beef Bourguignon, 87
Mushroom Ragu with Pappardelle, 98
Pasta Fagioli, 84
Red Lentil Bolognese with Creamy Polenta, 100

Cherries
Cherry-Cacao Shake (or Strawberry-Cacao Shake) , 9

Chick Peas
Chick Pea Lentil Balls, 86
Garlic Hummus, 37

Chives
Burrata Salad, 56
Creamy Cauliflower Soup, 54
Jalapeno Poppers (Vegetarian), 38

Cilantro
Mexican Street Corn on the Cob, 75

Corn
Arepas, 31
Creamy Parmesan Polenta, 100
Mexican Street Corn, 75

Cucumbers
Burrata Salad, 56
Collard Green Veggie Wraps with Seared Tofu, 76
Easy Homemade Pickles, 76
Mezze Platter, 36
Tzatziki Dip, 37

P.

Parsley
Mushroom Ragu with Pappardelle, 98
Shredded Chicken and Leek Soup, 50
Spicy Potatoes, 71

Peas, Sugar Snap
Crudité Platter, 45

Peppers
Black Bean and Sweet Potato Chili, 89
Collard Green Veggie Wraps with Seared Tofu, 76
Crudité Platter, 45
Vegetable Pancakes, 74
Quinoa and Black Bean Bake, 39

Pickles, Homemade
Collard Green Veggie Wraps with Seared Tofu, 76
Homemade Pickles, 76

Pineapple
Carrot Cake, 132

Potatoes, Japanese Sweet
Japanese Sweet Potato Loaf, 25

Potatoes, Sweet (or Yam)
Black Bean and Sweet Potato Chili, 89
Butternut Squash Soup, 55
Sweet Potato Gnocchi, 95

Potatoes, White (Russet)
Beef Bourguignon, 87
Potato Dumplings, 97
Vegetable Pancakes, 74

Potatoes, Yukon
Shredded Chicken and Leek Soup, 50
Spicy Potatoes, 71

Pomegranates
Burrata Salad, 56
Orange and Fennel Salad, 48

Pumpkin
Chai-Spiced Pumpkin Loaf, 16
Sweet Potato Gnocch, 95

R.

Radishes
Mezze Platter, 36

Raspberries
Raspberry Sauce, 124

S.

Sage
Butternut Squash Soup, 55

Shallots
Butternut Squash Soup, 55
Creamy Parmesan Polenta, 100
Shredded Chicken and Leek Soup, 50

Scallions
Carrot Fritters, 72
Dipping Sauce, 72
Quinoa and Black Bean Bake, 39
Spicy Asian-Inspired Crispy Cauliflower Bites with Honey-Chili Garlic Sauce, 61
Vegetable Pancakes, 74

Spinach
Green Matcha Shake, 8
Pesto Penne Pasta, 105

Strawberries
Strawberry-Cacao Shake, 9
Strawberry Oat Bites, 7

T.

Thyme
Beef Bourguignon, 87
Butternut Squash Soup, 55
Mini Goat Cheese and Prosciutto Pizzas, 41
Pasta Fagioli, 84

Tomatoes
End of Summer Harvest Green-Red Tomato Sauce, 94

Tomatoes, Canned
End of Summer Harvest Green-Red Tomato Sauce, 94
Mushroom Ragu with Pappardelle, 98
Red Lentil Bolognese with Creamy Parmesan Polenta, 100
Pasta Fagioli, 84

Y.

Yam
Japanese Yam Loaf, 25

Z.

Zucchini
Pasta Nerano, 103
Vegetable Pancakes, 74
Zucchini fritters, 73

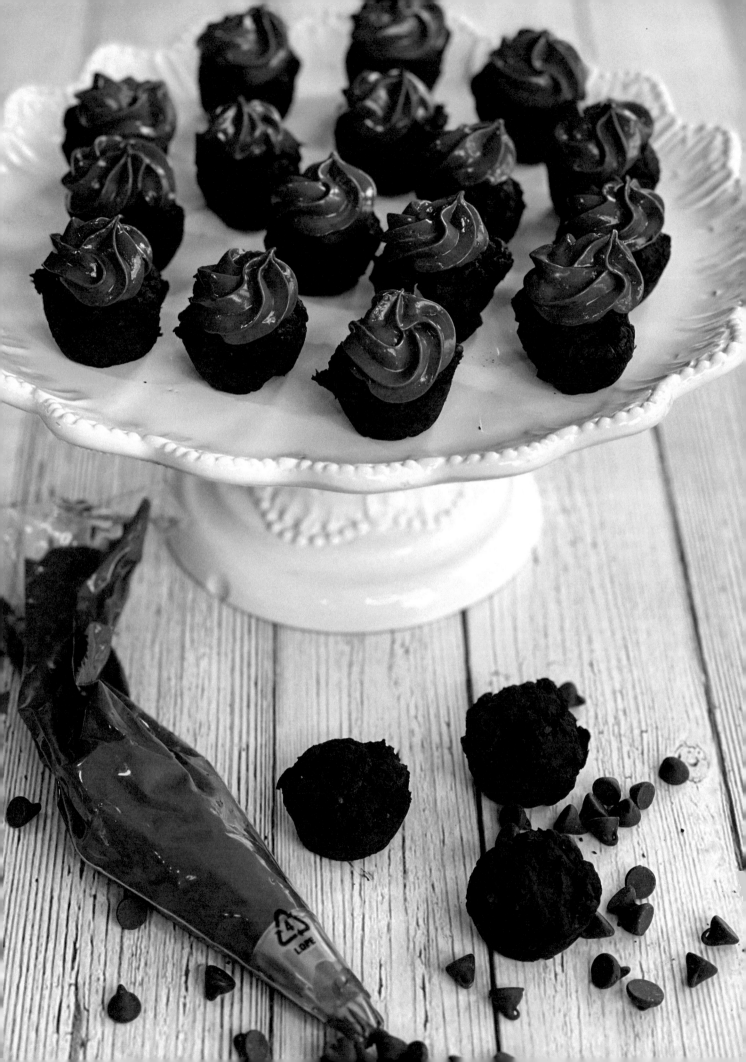